The Little Girl in the Radiator:
Mum, Alzheimer's and me

Martin Slevin

Monday Books

A CIP catalogue record for this title is available
from the British Library

ISBN: 978-1-906308-43-8

Typeset by Andrew Searle
Printed and bound by CPI Group (UK) Ltd,
Croydon, CR0 4YY

www.mondaybooks.com
http://mondaybooks.wordpress.com/
info@mondaybooks.com

Contents

Dedication

To my two children, Rebecca and Daniel, who just thought their grandmother was crazy but loved her anyway.

And to Heather, who helped me cope when no-one else could.

Also to all the family members of Alzheimer's patients out there; you're not alone.

To my Dad.

And lastly, but mostly, to my Mum.

All that follows is true.

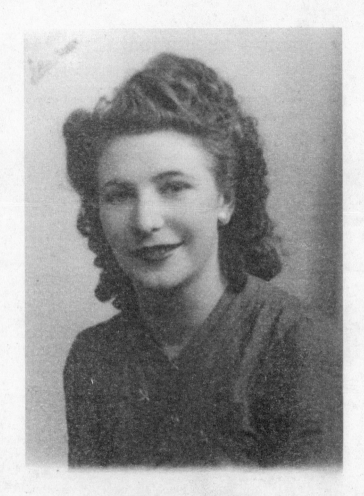

Rose Slevin, 1925-2007

Foreword

I should make it clear right at the outset that I have no formal medical training. I can stick a plaster on a cut finger, but that's about it. Everything I know about dementia, and about Alzheimer's disease in particular, I have either read in books or online or seen for myself at first-hand, as it were. The observations, comments, and conclusions I make throughout this book are my own.

In modern Britain, more money is spent on launching a new aftershave than on researching Alzheimer's disease; although we'd all like the male population to smell nice, I think we would also want our parents and grandparents to experience a quality of life during their dotage which is currently denied them through medical ignorance.

Some names and details of the care homes my mum went to have been changed for legal reasons, but the details of how she suffered in the first of them are absolutely accurate.

1. Rolling Up The Rug

ALZHEIMER'S DISEASE IS the only medical condition that I know of which affects the family of the patient more than it appears to affect the patient themselves.

The long tentacles of its colourful fantasies reach out in all directions at once, touching, clawing, caressing and embracing all who pass within their reach, until each is drawn into the labyrinthine tragedy and made to become an actor in the drama. While all of this is going on, the patient continues to move through their own little world, interacting with all of its colours, contours and characters as though nothing had happened or changed, blissfully unaware of the emotional turmoil they are causing in the outside universe.

If you break your leg, it incommodes you. *You* sit at home in plaster; *you* suffer and *you* deal with it: it's *your* problem. Your family members may be slightly inconvenienced, inasmuch as they will fetch and carry for you, but that's about the extent of their forced participation in your altered condition. With Alzheimer's, it's the other way around. If you have Alzheimer's disease, it becomes everyone else's problem; you behave as though nothing has changed, while everyone around you has to cope with your radically altered mentality.

'It's like rolling up a rug,' said the consultant. My mother and I were sitting in the Caludon Centre, at Coventry's Walsgrave Hospital, where she had been referred by her GP. He had suspected the onset of dementia when mum went to his surgery to complain about a little girl who was living inside a radiator at home, and who was whispering to her the most disturbing things about other members of our family. When the receptionist at the surgery heard this she had sent for the doctor, who had come out of his consulting room into the main waiting area to find mum causing mayhem among his other patients; she was climbing on one of the chairs and trying to take down his curtains, because they were too short and didn't reach the windowsill.

Now, the specialist looked across his desk at me and ignored my mum, who was sitting next to me, apparently unaware that she was being discussed at all.

'Imagine you're standing at one end of a long carpet,' he said. 'The end nearest to you represents the present, and the other end represents your mother's childhood. As we begin to roll up the rug, the memories inside the roll are erased and lost forever, and her reality slips backwards in time. The more we roll up the rug, the further back in time she has to travel to find a point in her life that she remembers.'

I nodded slowly, trying to understand. My mother looked at his burnt-orange curtains with a disgusted and professional eye. They were tatty and frayed, and had probably hung on the window for years. I knew she was thinking about how she could run up a much nicer pair for him in no time at all. In fact, I was waiting for her to ask him for the job.

'I want to ask your mother a few simple questions,' he said, finally looking at her.

She smiled back at him, amiably.

'What year is it now, Rose?'

My mother began to frown.

'Now that's a hard one,' she replied. 'Let me think. Is the war still on?'

The consultant smiled. 'Do you mean the Second World War?'

Mum nodded.

'No, that ended in 1945,' he said. 'What year is it now?'

'Then it must be after that,' she replied.

'It's 2002,' he said.

'Yes, that's right,' said mum, who would have agreed if he had said it was 1812, and Napoleon was running France.

I squeezed her hand gently, and she turned her head towards me and smiled.

'I am going to ask you to remember a few things, Rose,' he said, 'and then in a few minutes I will ask you to tell me what those things were. Is that okay?'

'Yes, that's okay,' said mum, looking back at him, and smiling.

'A pen, a newspaper, a pair of scissors, a clock and a pair of shoes,' he said slowly.

Mum nodded confidently.

'Who is the Prime Minister today?'

'Margaret Thatcher, the milk snatcher!' announced my mum, triumphantly.

As Minister for Education – before her election as Prime Minister of Britain in 1979 – Mrs Thatcher had been seen as being responsible for the ending of free school milk for Britain's children.

'No, it's Tony Blair at the moment,' replied the consultant.

'Oh, I see,' said mum. 'I don't like him.'

'What month is it?' asked the consultant.

'April!' said mum, with some certainty.

'No, it's August,' said the consultant.

'Yes, that's right,' said mum.

'Now, I want you to tell me, Rose, the list of items I gave you to remember a few minutes ago. Can you recall them?'

'Yes, I can,' she said. 'A pair of scissors.'

'Very good.' The consultant was nodding.

'A bicycle, a fur hat, and a box of chocolates!'

Mum looked very pleased with herself. The consultant had stopped nodding.

'I think we need to do some more tests,' he said.

* * * * *

There is no way of proving it now, but I am convinced that my mother's dementia began the day my father died. I believe the shock of his death somehow triggered the Alzheimer's condition in her.

My parents were married for over 50 years, and they were never apart during that time. Each was the other's right arm. My dad had undergone a triple heart bypass operation 15 years before; it gave him another decade and a half of life, but his health was broken. Slowly, very slowly, he had become an invalid; in the last year of my father's

11

life, my mother had nursed him like he was a sick child, and, even though it was seen coming a long way off, when death finally arrived she went into shock.

My parents were from Dublin; they had met and married there, and I was born in Ireland at a time when work and money were scarce. The family story goes that, in 1961, when I was four years old, the three of us were in the market in Dublin, and I asked for an apple. Mum rummaged through her purse and found she hadn't enough money.

'It's come to something when I can't even afford to buy my son a bloody apple!' said my dad, and within a week we had emigrated to Coventry. These days, like most places, it's struggling a little, but back then it was a thriving engineering city, the home of Jaguar cars – where my dad worked – Massey Ferguson tractors, the black London taxi and lots of other household names.

My mum was a talented seamstress, and she started a little business in our two-bedroomed bungalow, making curtains and matching bedspreads to order for people she knew. As word of her work spread, her orders increased, and my father built her an extension out into the back garden. This workroom was her world for the next 20 years: I can hardly recall a time when she wasn't back there, cutting, stitching, hand-sewing or measuring material. Hundreds of different coloured threads stuck out of the walls on little dowelling racks which my dad had made for her, and a long worktable and three industrial sewing machines completed her little factory. I mention my mother's sewing now as it explains her interest in her doctors' shabby old curtains, and becomes more relevant still later on.

The months leading up to and following my dad's death were difficult. During the same period, my own marriage was coming to an end, which was why I found myself, a year after he'd gone, sitting in my mum's kitchen and telling her I was going to move back in with her.

'Oh, that would be lovely!' she cried. 'But what about your wife, doesn't she mind?'

'We've split up,' I said, simply.

My mother looked at me vacantly; she didn't seem to understand what I was saying.

'Is she coming to stay, too?'

'No, we've separated, mum,' I said. 'We're going to get a divorce. Rebecca and Daniel will continue to live there, and I'll move back here. I mean, if that's all right with you?'

'That's great!' she announced. 'We can have tea together every day!'

For various reasons I'd not visited mum that often – once a week or so, and only then for a short while at a time – so I hadn't really seen the dementia ebbing and flowing through her mind like a slowly rising tide. But as I sat there, I realised that she was now noticeably worse than when we'd visited the consultant at the Caludon Centre a few months earlier. I moved back over the next day or two, filling the bedroom of my childhood with the remnants of my married life. Once I was ensconced, mum's decline quickly became more apparent to me.

I remember getting out of the shower one morning as I was preparing to go to work – at the time, I was a community warden for Coventry City Council. I stepped from the shower cubicle onto the mat in the bathroom and reached over to take a fresh towel from the rack. I was surprised when it just fell away into a series of perfectly cut strips – about 12 of them, all exactly the same width, each running the full length of the towel, and all laid back on the rack in perfect symmetry, one beside the other, like a row of soldiers on parade. As I would later learn, it is a characteristic trait of the victims of Alzheimer's disease, and dementia generally, that they continue obsessively to carry out once-familiar physical tasks, perhaps in an attempt to anchor themselves in the strange and unfamiliar new seas of their lives. In mum's mind, she was still at work, still cutting material to make curtains and bedding. It took me a long time to understand that.

'What's happened to this towel, mum?' I asked, standing in the hall naked and dripping with water, and holding up the perfect strips in either hand for my mother to see.

'I don't know,' she called back from the kitchen. 'What are you asking me for? It must have been Peggy. Ask her.'

'Peggy who?' I replied.

'Your aunt Peggy, of course,' she said. 'She's always doing things like that.'

'Mum,' I said, softly, 'Aunt Peggy's been dead for five years.'

'She is *not*!' insisted my mum. 'I spoke to her only yesterday. What are you saying things like that for?'

I thought about what the consultant had said... The rolling up of my mother's mental rug. If mum believed my aunt Peggy was still alive, then she must be living in a time at least five years in the past.

I found another towel.

* * * * *

Over the next two or three years, mum's decline was gradual, but inexorable. It wasn't just her mental faculties: she was fading away physically, too. I didn't notice this at first, but in late 2005 I suddenly realised that she was getting very thin.

She had always been petite, and had never put on weight despite having a good appetite. I think she lived on nervous energy most of her adult life – she never did fewer than three things at a time. She'd be out in her workroom making curtains or something, for instance, and would keep popping into the kitchen to peel a bowlful of potatoes for the family dinner, and dashing off a few lines of a letter to someone. (She was a compulsive letter writer, of which more later.) Then she would return to the workroom and carry on with her curtains. So she simply burned off whatever calories she consumed.

Now, I noticed, she was getting seriously thin. Clearly, I needed to get her eating properly. I decided to cook her a decent meal, and opened the cupboards to start rooting around for ingredients. Every packet, tin and box of food in the kitchen was months or even years out of date. She'd been less than assiduous in restocking the kitchen cupboards since my father had died.

'All this stuff is way past its best, mum,' I said, rummaging in a drawer for a roll of black bags.

She sat with her head in her hands and watched me empty all the old tins and packets into the bags for the bin men to collect on Thursday.

'You're going to starve me to death,' she sobbed. 'Wait until your father gets home. He'll have something to say about this!'

She used to say that to me when I had been a naughty child, and it still made me feel uncomfortable. Dad had always been the one to punish me, to stop my pocket money, to send me to my room. I suppose I was a handful as a kid, and I always seemed to be waiting for him to come home.

'You can't eat this stuff,' I said. 'Half of it would give you food poisoning.'

Mum shook her head. 'Your father won't be happy.'

'Dad's dead, mum,' I replied, bluntly. Too bluntly.

She looked at me with disgust in her eyes.

'How could you be so cruel as to say that to me? When I think of how much your father loves you, and all the things he does for you.'

'I know all that, mum, and I loved him too. But he's dead now, don't you understand that?'

The brutality of ignorance: later, much later, when I understood better how Alzheimer's worked, I was more tactful.

Mum simply continued to stare at me, shaking her head slowly from side to side in disbelief. 'Your father will be *very* angry with you when he gets home.'

I finished emptying the cupboards out, there was nothing left. I made a list of stuff we needed, and then turned to my mother.

'We have to go shopping now, mum,' I said. 'It's cold outside, put a coat on.'

Like an obedient child, she rose from the kitchen table and went into the hall. She took a pale beige belted raincoat from the closet and put it on. It should have reached down to her knees, but as she stood there in the hallway I saw that it ended at her waist. Underneath the beltline it was all tattered; it had been cut in half.

'I'm ready,' she said.

'What happened to your coat?' I sighed.

'Peggy shortened it for me,' she said.

I took a deep breath. 'You can't wear that,' I replied.

I went into her bedroom and removed another coat from her wardrobe. 'Put this one on,' I said, handing it to her, without looking at it too much.

'You're being very bossy with me today,' replied mum. She took off the half-a-raincoat and dropped it on the floor, slipping on the other in its place. It was a dark blue cashmere affair; I remembered my father buying it one year for her birthday.

'Now can we go?' she said.

The stitching around the left shoulder seam of the blue coat had been unpicked and the sleeve removed.

'For Christ's sakes, mother!' I exclaimed.

'What's the matter now?' she shouted.

'It's only got one fucking sleeve!' I screamed.

'Don't you dare swear at me!' she yelled back. 'You wait until your father gets home!'

'Dad's fucking dead!' I bellowed.

Mum ran into her bedroom and threw herself down on her bed, sobbing louder and harder than I can ever remember. I stood in the hall feeling like a complete shit. I went into her bedroom and held her in my arms, and we cried together.

Eventually we stood up, and I went back to her wardrobe. I took out another coat, checked to see that it was okay, and got her to put that one on. It was bright green, it didn't match anything she was wearing, but I didn't care. At least it was intact.

'Peggy must have taken the sleeve off the blue one,' said mum. 'She's a bitch for doing that, isn't she?'

We drove to Tesco and parked the car.

'Can we buy some cream cakes and chocolate biscuits?' asked mum brightly, seeming to have forgotten the events back at the house.

'Sure we can,' I replied. 'We can buy whatever you want.'

She beamed at me.

It was Saturday morning, a cold, late November day, and Christmas was only a month away. The supermarket was packed with shoppers, and the shelves were stacked with fancy Christmas knick-knacks. Mum was like a little girl again. In the centre of the store stood a huge Christmas tree with tinsel and streamers all around its splayed branches. Hundreds of little fairy lights winked magically on and off.

'That's so beautiful,' observed my mother, standing and gazing at the tree. 'I wish we had a tree like that.'

'We will have,' I replied. 'I'll put our tree up in a week or so, we can decorate it together.'

She opened her mouth wide with delight.

'Can we really?' she gasped.

I nodded.

Suddenly, unexpectedly, she hugged me. Mum had never really been one for hugs, and it took me by surprise.

We started to shop for tinsel and cream cakes. Mum would see a chocolate éclair and put it in the trolley. Then we would move on to another aisle, suddenly she would rush back and get another cream cake.

'Just in case,' she would say, putting the extra one in the trolley.

We wandered around Tesco that morning stocking up on all the healthy stuff: chocolate biscuits, chocolate bars, jam sponges, éclairs, jam doughnuts, and ice cream. I think we bought one or two bits of the boring stuff as well, for form's sake – a chicken and some potatoes come to mind – but they were more of an afterthought.

'This is lovely!' declared mum, as we wandered about. I had not seen her this happy in ages.

When we came to the Christmas decorations she really went to town, strewing tinsels of a dozen glittering hues around our shopping trolley. She found an illuminated pair of plastic elf ears, and put them on. She looked like Mr Spock on acid as we bustled through the busy supermarket. She was clearly having the time of her life.

'You didn't tell me it was Christmas,' she said. 'I haven't bought anyone a present yet.'

'We can sort that out later,' I replied, hoping she would forget about it. The thought of buying presents for all our dead relatives didn't really appeal to me.

Mum nodded thoughtfully and pressed on through the busy aisles, totally heedless of the amused glances she was drawing from passers-by, her elf ears flashing like mad as she went.

2. The Eternal Christmas Tree

THE NEXT FEW weeks were idyllic. Mum was very well into the festive spirit, and each afternoon I would return from work and be met at the door with a beaming smile, and the same question: 'Is it Christmas yet?'

But a couple of incidents left a sour taste in my mouth. Alzheimer's patients lose their grounding in time (as their rug is continually rolled up); as a result, they're often confused and become very suggestible. This makes them vulnerable to unscrupulous salesmen.

I came home one afternoon to find the house looking like it had been hit by a tornado. Bits of the front fascia and guttering were spread across the lawn, a ladder was propped against the roof and a young man of around 20 years of age was busy ripping down the rest of the gutters with a crowbar. His mate stood in the front garden, throwing the debris onto the back of a flat-bed truck.

'What the hell's going on here?' I asked.

'The old lady's having new soffits, fascias and guttering,' replied the man on the ground.

'The hell she is!' I shouted. 'Come down from there!'

The two men stood next to me in the garden.

'Who gave you permission to do this?' I said.

The lad who had been on the roof seemed to be in charge. 'The old lady did,' he said.

'Wait here, and don't do anything else,' I said. 'By the way, how much do you think you're charging her?'

'What's it to you?' he said.

'I'm her son,' I replied, 'and "the old lady", as you call her, happens to be my mother. She also has Alzheimer's disease, and can't tell you what day of the week it is. *I* decide what needs to be done around here. It's me that pays the money.'

'She's already agreed it,' said the one in charge.

'That makes no difference,' I said. 'How much?'

'Two thousand, five hundred pounds,' came the reply. He said the figure so casually he made it sound like two pounds and fifty pence.

'*How* much?' I shouted. 'We'll see about this!'

I went storming into the house.

'Is it Christmas yet?' asked mum, beaming. She was wearing the flashing elf ears.

'Who are those men in the garden?' I asked, trying to ignore the ears.

'I don't know,' replied mum. 'Who are they?'

'They're tearing the roof off the house!' I shouted. 'They say you've agreed to pay them two and a half thousand pounds. The roof is perfectly fine, it doesn't need replacing.'

Mum shrugged her shoulders. 'I don't know,' she said. 'Maybe it was Peggy.'

I picked up the telephone and dialled enquiries. 'Trading Standards for Coventry, please.'

They gave me the number. I spoke to a Trading Standards officer who told me they had received a number of complaints in the area regarding rogue traders. I told him what had happened. As luck would have it, he said, one of their officers was in the area dealing with another incident. They would call him and ask him to visit me next. I gave them our address.

'Did you sign anything?' I asked mum.

'Like what?'

'Like a contract of any kind. A piece of paper, anything. Did you sign your name on anything for those men outside?' I was nearly hysterical.

'I don't know,' came back the standard response. 'Ask Peggy.'

I went back outside.

'Right,' I said to the two men, who had stopped work and were waiting for me. 'Let me explain something to you. My mother has a disease called Alzheimer's. It affects the brain. People with it are very confused and suggestible. It also means that they cannot enter into any sort of legal contract because they are not of sound mind.

Therefore any contract she has with you is not enforceable at law, so I suggest you pack up your stuff and leave right now.'

They looked at each other. 'We need paying for our work,' announced the one in charge.

'You're not getting a penny,' I said. 'In fact, I should have you both for criminal damage.'

'We've got a contract!' piped up the other. He pulled a single sheet of paper from the inside pocket of his jacket and handed it to me. It was an A4 sheet which had obviously been produced on a home computer. It was full of spelling mistakes, bad grammar and had no business address anywhere on the sheet. At the bottom was my mother's signature.

'This is useless,' I said, handing it back to him. 'It's not a legal contract.'

'Yes it is!' said the other one. 'We're doing the work that the old lady asked us to do! If you want us to stop now, that's okay, but we need paying for our time up to now.'

'My mother didn't ask you to do anything,' I replied. 'You have taken advantage of her. You told her the work needed doing, which it did not. She didn't understand what you were saying, and simply agreed because she's suggestible. She doesn't even remember signing that, and doesn't know what the work is for anyway.'

'We can settle this in court, if you like,' said the one in charge.

Feeling this was his final threat, I decided to call his bluff. 'Fine. Let's do that,' I agreed. 'Let's take it to court. And I'll stand up and tell the judge that you coerced an 80-year-old lady with Alzheimer's disease to have unnecessary work done to her house, so you could charge her two and a half thousand pounds. You'll be lucky if you both don't end up in prison.'

They looked at each other; suddenly, they didn't seem so sure of their ground.

A car pulled up outside the house, and a dark-suited man got out. He walked up the front path and joined us. He pulled a wallet from his jacket and showed it to all three of us.

'Trading Standards,' he said.

I watched the two lads visibly pale. 'Thanks for coming,' I said.

He smiled at me. 'What's the problem?' he asked.

'He won't pay us for the work we've done,' said the one in charge, before I had a chance to speak.

'We've got a contract with the old lady,' chimed in the other. He held the single sheet of paper out to the Trading Standards officer, who took it and read it slowly.

Without a word he refolded the paper and handed it back.

'Is the homeowner inside the house?' he asked me.

'She is,' I replied.

'I need to speak to her,' he said, and headed towards the front door.

Like three schoolchildren not sure if we were in trouble or not, we trooped in silence behind him up the garden path.

He rang the bell. I just knew what would happen next.

Mum opened the door, resplendent in a new one-sleeved cardigan, odd slippers, and flashing ears.

'Hello,' she said, with quiet dignity.

'Hello, Mrs Slevin,' said the man, 'I am from Trading Standards. May I come in and have a word?'

Mum retreated back into the house, and he entered. Just as he shut the door behind him, we all heard mum ask him quietly, 'Is it Christmas yet?'

The three of us stood staring at each other in silence. Around our feet lay the shattered remains of the guttering and fascia boards from the front of mum's house. I wondered what my dad would have said.

'We've got a contract you know,' said one of them.

'We'll see,' I replied.

The door opened and the Trading Standards chap came out.

'You two gentlemen seem to have a problem,' he said quietly. 'I'm sure you're both aware that there are certain sections of the community with whom you cannot by law enter into a legal contract. Minors, for instance. Anyone under the age of 18 cannot enter into any agreement enforceable at law; neither can anyone of unsound mind, a mental patient, whether they are institutionalised or not.

This lady has been medically diagnosed with Alzheimer's disease, and therefore is of unsound mind. She cannot be a party to a legal agreement without her official carer's consent and approval. In short, gentlemen, the paper you have is worthless.'

I breathed a sigh of relief.

The other two looked at each other and shrugged their shoulders.

'What about the work we've already done today?' asked the one in charge.

'That work was not properly and legally authorised,' he replied. 'Therefore, technically, you have damaged the property. But that's something for you and the homeowner's legal guardian to sort out between yourselves.'

'I'm not paying a penny!' I said. I knew there was little hope of getting *them* to pay *me*.

Eventually, with much muttering and grumbling, they packed up their gear and left. The front of the property still looked like NATO had been testing rockets on it.

'I know a professional builder who can put this right for you,' said the officer. 'I'll give you his number.'

A few days later the house was as good as new, though it cost me £650 to repair the damage. I thought about suing the two men, but it transpired they were working out of a flat, had no savings, no proper credentials or qualifications and no insurance.

It was an expensive lesson – that, sadly, there are people who have absolutely no regard for the dignity or rights of others, especially if those others are weak or vulnerable. It was a lesson I was to learn over and over again. (In fact, it was one of the reasons I decided to write this book – to raise awareness of the Alzheimer's patient's vulnerability. If they are to live in the community, then some consideration must be made for this vulnerability; they and their carers must be protected by the law to a greater extent than they are at present.)

* * * * *

Christmas got closer, and it was time for me to keep my promise to mum, and put up the old tree. It was a six foot tall, artificial thing which my dad had dutifully dragged out of the loft, year after year, for as long as I could remember. It came in three separate sections which slotted together and then fitted into a plastic base; I remember dad carefully assembling it each year, before standing back, shaking his head sadly and swearing that we'd get a new one in time for next Christmas.

I assembled the thing fairly quickly, and found myself unconsciously imitating my dad, with a shake of my own head. It had probably looked quite good in around 1975; now, though, it was so bedraggled that it was fit only for a skip. Half of the little green plastic spines were missing and its branches and bits of metal frame poked out at the most bizarre and unrealistic angles from the disintegrating trunk; it looked like no tree on earth.

It occurred to me that it was as eccentric as my mother – who was wearing her nightie under a new one-sleeved cardigan – and as worn out and frayed at the edges as I was.

'Oh, that's beautiful!' she cried, clapping her hands together in genuine delight. 'We must decorate it straight away.'

'There's a box of tinsel and some glass baubles in the loft,' I said. 'I'll get them.'

But when I returned from the loft I found she had already started. She was dancing around in front of the tree with a roll of Andrex in one hand; with the other, she was ripping off great streamers and casting them gaily across the plastic branches. The tree was already barely visible beneath a shroud of randomly-placed strips of pink loo roll.

'That's nice, mum,' I said.

'Do you like it?' she asked innocently, and stood back to admire her handiwork. 'Personally, I think it needs some lights.'

We hung glass baubles on the branches, and we wound an old set of fairy lights that I'd found in the attic around it. I switched them on, and mum squealed like a little girl with the pure, innocent delight of it all.

'It's so lovely!' she cried, performing a little dance in front of the oddest Christmas tree in the whole world.

I was expecting the lights to set fire to the toilet paper at any moment; I couldn't take my eyes off it.

'We must invite some people around to look at our tree,' said mum. 'What about Mary next door?'

The elderly, wheelchair-bound lady who lived next door had been a good friend to my mother. We had become firm friends ourselves, too – she had telephoned me at work at least twice a week for the last few months to tell me that mum had locked herself out of the house, and could I possibly come home and let her back in? She also saw more clearly than I did the truth of mum's position.

'She shouldn't be left on her own when you go to work,' she had said firmly to me one day. 'She can't be trusted on her own. She could fall asleep and leave the cooker on. She could have an accident, anything could happen. You need some help.'

She meant putting mum into a home; I knew she was right but I just didn't want to think about it.

'Er… Mary's asleep right now,' I said. 'We'll ask her over tomorrow.'

As soon as mum went to bed that night, I took all the pink toilet paper off the tree, and replaced it with the coloured tinsel we had bought at Tesco. The tree still looked a little bizarre, but then it would, I thought to myself, as I switched off the lights.

The next morning I went to work at 7am. Mum was still asleep. When I came home at 4.30pm, she had obviously had a busy day decorating the rest of the house. The first thing I noticed was one of my socks pinned to the wallpaper in the hallway. This was not a Christmas stocking, you understand, like one you might hang over the fireplace for the kids; it was an ordinary blue sock, stuck right in the middle of the wall with a simple dress-maker's pin. I stared at it for ages, then went in and shut the door behind me. Inside, I saw that just about every sock I possessed was pinned up – some to the walls and others to the ceiling. Even a brown one with a hole in the toe, which I had been meaning to throw out, was there.

Mum danced into the hall. 'I've been putting up the decorations!' she cried, with a majestic sweep of her arms. 'We're going to have a wonderful Christmas!'

'I can see you've been busy,' I agreed.

'Peggy helped me,' she said, matter-of-factly.

'Good for Peggy,' I sighed. 'Are you hungry?'

'I am *starving*!' replied mum. 'I haven't had a thing to eat all day long!'

'I'll make us something,' I said, taking my coat off, and wondering what I was going to use for socks tomorrow morning.

When I went into the kitchen, the fridge door was wide open and its entire contents were strewn across the floor. Bottles of milk, lumps of cheese, salad stuffs, butter. The fridge itself was empty, except for two slices of bread lying side by side on one of the empty shelves.

'What's all this?' I asked.

'I've been waiting all day for that bloody toaster to work,' said mum, ruefully.

We stared into the empty fridge together, at the two slices of bread.

'We'll have to get a new one,' said mum, shaking her head.

'You go inside and watch some television,' I said. 'I'll get the dinner ready.'

I put the contents of the fridge back, and threw out the now-stale bread. Then I opened the oven door, took out two pairs of mum's shoes, put them away, and turned it on.

I am not a good cook. I can do a fairly basic meat-and-two-veg, at a push, but nothing fancy. I put some oven chips in and cracked some eggs into a pan. Suddenly there was a scream from the front room.

I ran next door to find mum hiding behind a cushion.

'That thing has just gobbled up that poor little boy!' she screamed, the tears rolling down her cheeks.

I looked where she was pointing: *Jaws* was on telly.

'It's okay, mum,' I said, putting my arm around her. 'It's just a film.'

26

She was genuinely upset. 'They shouldn't let things like that get into the swimming pool!' she cried, now indignant. 'I'm going to write a letter to the council!'

This was the beginning of our letter-writing period.

'Okay, mum,' I said, taking the remote control. 'Let's watch something else.'

I changed the channel over to cartoons. Jerry the cat was being chased around the kitchen, and was being whacked over the head with an old-fashioned broomstick.

'That's better,' I said, 'you watch that.'

Mum's tears quickly turned to laughter. I could hear her still laughing as I returned to the kitchen. She enjoyed a good cartoon as much as any child ever did.

On the kitchen table there was a dishcloth and a pair of scissors. I held up the dishcloth, it had a perfect circle cut out of the middle of it. The circle was pinned to the wallpaper, complete with some unidentifiable brown stain in the middle of it. Next to it was a square cut out of another towel. The towel had been replaced on the rail by the sink. I didn't bat an eyelid. It's funny; you get used to almost anything.

Simple egg-and-chips later, we sat together watching cartoons. Mum laughed out loud, and her laughter, always being infectious, made me laugh, too. But as I sat there, I couldn't escape a strange feeling that was nagging away at me. *Something* was different in the room, I had known that as soon as I sat down – I just couldn't say what it was. With half an eye on Daffy Duck, I looked around. Twenty-odd socks pinned to the wallpaper and the ceiling... Yep, that was all as expected. Two cut-up towels draped over the arm of the chair: yep, all normal, (for our house, anyway). I couldn't put my finger on it. Then it hit me.

'What's happened to the door?' I yelped, leaping out of the chair.

'The man came and changed it,' said mum, casually.

'What man?' I shouted.

When I'd left for work that morning the door between the living room and the conservatory my father had built years ago had been a fairly modest affair – wooden, very plain and painted white. Now, I saw, it had been replaced by a huge, brown, sliding, uPVC thing, with faux leaded lights criss-crossing the window panes in small diamonds.

'*What* man?' I repeated, touching the door, and sliding it back and forth to make sure it was real. Up close, I could see that the plasterwork around the frame was new and freshly painted, too. This would not have been cheap.

'The man who came and changed the door, of course,' said mum. 'Sit down, I can't see the television.'

It may sound like a contradiction in terms, but when you live with someone who has Alzheimer's you get used to being surprised. The most bizarre things suddenly happen, and yet you take them in your stride as though they were an everyday occurrence in every home in the land. But I must admit that this change in the back wall of the living room, all in the few hours since I had left for work that morning, had thrown me a bit.

'But…but…' I stammered, trying to work out how I could possibly get to the bottom of this with only mum to supply the answers.

'Shh!' she replied, impatiently waving me away from in front of the screen.

'How much money did the man ask you for?' I asked, timidly.

'He didn't ask me for anything,' replied mum.

'Well, did he leave you any paperwork?' I asked.

'I don't think so. Ask Peggy.'

'Did you know the man?' I was now clutching at straws.

Mum shook her head slowly. 'He looked a bit like Richard.'

'Uncle Richard?' I asked.

'Mmm, but a lot shorter.'

This was getting me nowhere. I began to search the kitchen for an invoice, an estimate for the work, a business card. I couldn't find anything.

A few days later a bill for £4,000 arrived in the post. I nearly fainted when I opened the envelope, but at least I could begin to piece the jigsaw together. It seemed that, a few weeks ago, a double-glazing salesman had called to the house while I was at work. Mum had agreed to his suggestions and signed the work order, and promptly forgot all about it. When the workman turned up to do the job, mum just let him get on with it. She liked him and trusted him, because he looked a bit like Uncle Richard (only shorter), and when he had gone away mum had forgotten all about that, too.

I telephoned the company. I was on the line for about 20 minutes; I won't bore you with the details of each conversation I had with the receptionist, the sales department, the works department, and the accounts department, and the supervisors of each of those; suffice it to say that I got pretty much nowhere. I tried to explain to them, as I had to the two men in our front garden a few weeks previously, that my mother was not able to enter into a legal contract, and therefore could not be held accountable for the order they had received from her, as she didn't understand it. They all simply insisted that due process had been followed, the works order had been signed by the customer, she had been given two weeks to change her mind, and since she had not returned her form to cancel the order the work had been carried out; now we owed them the money. In frustration, I eventually hung up.

I felt as though my mother had again been violated in some way by a system that took no notice of her obvious condition. I felt violated for her… I felt angry and used; it was almost as though she had been mugged in the street. In the end I simply scrawled across the invoice 'WORK NOT LEGALLY REQUESTED' and sent it back to the firm.

When you deal with large organisations whose paperwork is primarily generated by a computer, the human element seems to get mislaid somewhere in the mix. The following week, I received the same invoice again, and I returned it in the same way. Christmas came and went, and the requests for the money, and my rejection of the invoices flew back and forth between us like a tennis ball. Eventually, a notice of court proceedings dropped onto the doormat around February. Below is my reply. The letter has not been changed at all, except that I omit my mother's address and the name of the company concerned for obvious reasons.

Dear Sir,

It seems I have to write to you to explain in plain and simple language what your sales representative should have been able to see with his own eyes.

The lady with whom you state you have a sales contract is in fact an 80 year-old Alzheimer's patient, living at home, and completely unable to comprehend the terms or implications of such a contract. Because she is not 'compos mentis' she is not held responsible in law for the terms of any contract she enters into. In fact, I, as her son, have her sole Power of Attorney for exactly that reason, so that any legal contracts have to be agreed and signed by me in order for them to become binding on her; I have given no such consent at any time to your company.

If you wish to pursue this matter further through the courts, then I suggest you prepare yourself and your company to be portrayed in the public press as the kind of outfit that browbeats elderly, defenceless mental patients into parting with their life savings for home improvements they neither need nor require.

I look forward to hearing from you in due course,

Yours faithfully,

Martin Slevin.

We never heard from them again, and I felt I had achieved a little victory for Alzheimer's patients and their families everywhere.

That said, I must admit that it was a very nice door.

3. The Little Girl In The Radiator

ON THE MONDAY BEFORE that Christmas, I came home from work to find mum sitting in one armchair in the living room watching television, and a great featherless and headless bird sitting in the other armchair, as though watching the box with her.

It had been positioned in the armchair the right way up, so that its enormous, drumstick legs pointed down, and it was resting with its back against a cushion facing the TV screen. It had been placed there while frozen, but it had begun to thaw out and a great wet patch was now spreading out behind and below it across the fabric of the chair.

'What's this, mum?' I asked, expecting her to explain to me how some long lost relative had come to stay with us for Christmas, or something like that.

'It's our Christmas turkey, of course,' she replied, as though I was an idiot. 'I got him from the supermarket this morning. I couldn't resist him. Isn't he smashing?'

There was a paper tag on one of the creature's legs which announced proudly:

> GIANT CHRISTMAS GOOSE.
> WILL FEED TWELVE PEOPLE.

The damned thing was the size of a Rottweiler.

'How the hell did you get it home?' I asked, struggling under the weight of the mighty bird as I hauled its frozen carcass off the armchair.

'A man gave me a lift back,' she said.

'What man?' I asked.

'He looked like your Uncle Bernard,' replied mum. 'Only fatter.'

A feeling of *déjà vu* swept over me. Her eyes never moved from the television screen.

'Never mind,' I sighed. I wasn't going through all that again.

I hauled the huge goose into the kitchen and threw it onto the floor. It landed with a sloppy splat like some sort of suicidal nudist, with splinters of ice flying up into the air. I looked at our small fridge. Shaking my head, I knelt down and took out most of the contents and two shelves. I could just about get the goose in now, but I couldn't shut the door. I sat back and sighed. I'd not expected to spend the evening wrestling with a headless 25lb bird. Like I said, it's amazing what you get used to.

I hauled it out again, put the fridge back together and wondered what to do next. Christmas Day was still nearly a week off, and unless I could cold-store this thing somewhere it wouldn't be fit to eat. I checked our small freezer: it was also full. (I established this by quickly pulling out the three drawers, one after the other, seeing they were stacked, and shoving them closed again, without examining their contents. Only later did I discover it was actually packed with 50 packets of chocolate biscuits; but that's another story.)

I thought about the people I knew who might have a fridge large enough to take a giant goose, but I couldn't think of anyone. I began to walk about the house looking here and there for inspiration, and found myself in the garage. Like so many people, we never put our car in there, even through the harshest winters; instead, we left it sitting all night in the street, and filled the garage instead with a lifetime's collection of useless junk and worthless memorabilia. My old school reports (must try harder), rolls of carpet (must get this cleaned), a mostly cracked, china dinner service (must glue this all back together one day), my dad's tools (you never know when you'll need an Allen key), the lawnmower we no longer needed after dad had paved the lawn...

Dad's tools! I spun around and spied his old saw; it was a bit rusty now, but if I sawed the goose into quarters, perhaps people would be able to store it for me then? I picked up the rusty saw and waved it about me like it was Excalibur. Then a little voice in my head told me I would probably poison the both of us if I used it on the bird. Back to the drawing board.

32

It was bitterly cold at night that winter…

A few moments later I stood back and admired my ingenuity. The goose was sitting on a wooden garden chair next to a small round garden table. We used to take our meals out there in the summer. It could sit outside, the temperature would be cold enough and the meat wouldn't go off; it was too big for a stray cat to drag away in the middle of the night. I smiled: another problem solved.

* * * * *

After supper in the evenings, mum and I would watch television together and chat. I remember our talks together as being some of the nicest times we shared, even if the conversations were a bit off the wall.

She would tell me all the events of her day, while I had been at work – about the cowboys on their magnificent horses who had driven great herds of cattle past our window as they went up the street, about the burning plane that had crashed in our front garden, and about the great ship that had sunk in the middle of the road outside.

At first, I thought these stories were simply the Alzheimer's sharpening her imagination, and presenting her with fascinating delusions. Later – after the *Jaws* incident – I realised she was only relating to me whatever she had been watching on the television earlier in the day. The cowboys were from an old western movie, the plane crash from a war film, the ship was the *Titanic*, and so on. When she watched a movie she lost the ability to separate fact from fiction, and the events of those films became real to her, as though they had actually played out for real, in the street outside, or even inside the house itself. It got to the point where I would listen carefully to her account of the events of her day and then try to guess the film she had been watching. After she had gone to bed, I'd check the TV listings in the paper; I was right more than once.

It is terribly emotionally draining to watch the daily mental deterioration of a person you have loved all of your life. It's like witnessing a daily robbery, where each time another precious piece of their mind is stolen, and no matter what steps you take it can never be recovered. It's irreversible: once it's gone, it's gone. To watch a once-keen and sharp mind become steadily confused and blunted, to witness mental dexterity disappear like the water from a leaking pot, tears your soul in two. The anger and frustration you feel as a helpless bystander to this awful crime leaves you in shreds.

We were watching TV after supper one evening, and mum leaned over and looked at the radiator which ran the length of the back wall of the living room. I watched as she smiled lovingly at it, and nodded once or twice. Her lips moved as though she were saying something, and then she nodded her head again. Then she looked back at the television. I had seen her do this before but had never remarked upon it. Whereas in a healthy person it would have caused a mild alarm, with mum it was almost insignificant. But her attention to the radiator had been growing in frequency as the weeks had passed, and I thought I needed to say something.

'What are you doing, mum?' I asked, gently.

Her cheeks flushed red in embarrassment, and she shook her head but did not reply: she looked as though she had been caught doing something she shouldn't, something that was to be kept secret even from me.

'What's wrong with the radiator?' I asked.

'Nothing,' she said.

'Then why are you talking to it?' I said, trying not to make the question sound like an interrogation.

She shook her head again, and said nothing.

We continued to watch television that night, programme after programme. Out of the corner of my eye I would secretly watch her move her head ever so slightly towards the radiator, and smile. She would whisper something I couldn't hear, and then suddenly turn back to the TV if she thought I was watching. It became a game between us: could she talk secretly to the radiator more times than I could catch her?

In the end I had to get to the bottom of this.

'Why don't you tell me what's going on with the radiator, mum?' I asked.

She shook her head again.

'Go on, tell me. I won't tell anyone else,' I whispered. I think by now this radiator game had become a fascinating battle of wills.

'She's asked me not to!' exclaimed mum, with tears filling her eyes. 'When you give your word to someone, you should always try and keep it.'

'Who's asked you not to say anything?' I said.

Again she shook her head.

'You can tell me, mum,' I urged.

'The little girl in the radiator,' she said.

I thought about this for a moment.

'Why doesn't she want you to tell anyone?'

After a long silence, in which mum seemed to be weighing a problem in her mind, she turned away from the television to face me.

'Because she's all alone in there,' she said, the tears springing from her eyes. 'She's trapped and she's frightened, and I don't know how to help her.'

I went across the room and put my arm around her. She sobbed into my shoulder.

'What can I do to help?' I whispered.

'You're not supposed to know,' she sobbed.

'Tell her you've told me,' I said, 'and tell her I can be trusted not to tell anyone else. Tell her I might be able to help.'

Mum nodded and wiped her eyes, but continued to face the television. Then I saw her turn her head, and have a long conversation with the little girl in the radiator. I pretended not to notice. Then she turned back to me.

'She says it's all right for you to know,' said mum, quietly.

'That's good,' I said. 'How can I help her?'

'You could let her out!' cried mum, and the tears came again.

'Tell her, I said it's okay, she can come out,' I replied.

We hugged again.

Mum put her hand on the lukewarm radiator and began to whisper to the little girl trapped in there.

Eventually she looked back at me. 'It's not that simple,' she whispered.

It's funny how easily you can get caught up in another person's delusion, especially if you happen to live with them. After that night, I found myself talking to the little girl in the radiator with mum on many occasions. We would have three-way conversations, mum, the little girl and I, although the little girl never once spoke directly to me, always addressing me through mum.

I have no idea whether this practice was good for my mother's mental wellbeing or not. A psychiatrist might say that I was strengthening the delusion by playing along with it, but what was my alternative? If I told mum there was no little girl living inside the radiator, that a child could not possibly be trapped inside a hot water system two inches wide, she would have thought I was either too blind to see or too insensitive to care; the delusions of Alzheimer's do not require logic in order to grip their owner and hold them fast. The little girl *was* trapped in there, and mum had agreed to help her; if I was to help mum, then I had to join in too. To do otherwise would have driven a wedge between us, and that was something I did not want to risk; this way, at least, we were able to share our time together. So together, we spoke every night to the little girl in the radiator, and slowly over the following weeks, the little girl's sad and pitiful history began to unfold.

Mum went to bed around nine-thirty that particular night, which was very early for her. She said that talking to the little girl in the radiator had tired her, and made her upset. It was a terrible thing to be so cruel to a child, she said, and she couldn't understand how anyone could do such a thing.

I watched some more telly, and then surfed the internet for an hour or so, chatting online with friends. When I felt sleepy, I began my nightly inspection of the house before retiring. I made sure all the windows were closed, and locked the front door. I stood on a chair to take down a pair of socks from the woollen forest festooning the living room ceiling to wear tomorrow for work, and I looked out into the back garden and made sure the goose was still sitting in the garden chair.

It was there: everything was normal.

4. The Irish Band

I CAN'T REMEMBER exactly when the Irish band moved in.

I do know that there were at least six of them. There was an accordion player, at least one guitarist, a fiddle player and a banjo player. There was also a singer called Michael, who had a beautiful voice, according to mum. I suppose I was very grateful to the lads in those days, for they kept her amused for hours with their foot-tapping Irish tunes, and I know she enjoyed listening to them and singing along.

The band also kept her away from the TV, so she didn't get nearly as upset as she had done, and she was confident that they would be a great source of entertainment over Christmas dinner. Even the little girl who lived in the radiator liked the band (I think she had a thing for Michael), and mum said it was the happiest she had ever known her.

It was the day before Christmas Eve, and the nine of us were all getting along famously.

My decision to play along with mum's delusions meant that I had to participate in a practical sense, too. My mum, being Irish, loved her cups of tea, and would never make one just for herself. Whenever she fancied a cup she made one for each member of the band as well, and one also for the little girl in the radiator (or, more often, a glass of milk). There was also a cup for me. It was the same for sandwiches while I was at work. I would often come home to find every cup and plate in the house in use; with at least eight cold cups of tea scattered around the living room and kitchen, a glass of milk by the radiator, and numerous plates of uneaten sandwiches lying here and there.

When the house was crowded, as it was that Christmas, we were going through a loaf of bread and three pints of milk every single day, not to mention all the chocolate biscuits.

One Saturday morning I had arranged to walk down to the pub to have a drink with my mate, Andrew. We didn't see each other that often, but it was nice to have a pint together now and then and catch up. I took the last of the cash I had in the house, around £30 I think, and began to walk down the road. I left mum in the house listening to *I'll Take You Home Again Kathleen* (sung so beautifully by Michael that mum was almost in tears), and went to meet Andrew. On the way to the pub I called into Harry's for a packet of cigarettes.

Harry's was a small corner shop where you could buy just about anything, about halfway between our house and the nearest pub. Harry was an Indian chap who had been running the place for as long as anyone in the area could remember, and he knew every single one of his customers by name, knew who they were related to, knew what they liked and didn't like, and was always ready with a smile and a joke for anyone who entered his little shop. With Harry, you got such a personal service that everyone went to him, but despite this he was fighting a defensive battle against the advance of the giant supermarkets.

'Hi, Martin!' he called as I entered his shop, the familiar little brass bell tinkling over my head.

He reached behind him for my brand of cigarettes.

'Hi, Harry,' I said.

I put my hand in my pocket to pay for the smokes.

'That's £58.60 please, Martin,' he said, handing over the packet of 20 cigarettes.

I looked at him as though he had just gone mad.

'You what?' I gasped.

'Your mum was in here yesterday,' explained Harry. 'She took all the chocolate biscuits I had. She cleaned me out. Fifty packets! Then she just walked out. I didn't want to say anything, because I know she's not been herself lately, and because I knew you'd be in in a couple of days.'

'Didn't you think that 50 packets of chocolate biscuits was a bit excessive, Harry?' I asked, slapping my last £30 down on the counter, my pint with Andrew receding from view.

'Well, I suppose so,' he admitted, 'but it's not really up to me to tell people what they can, and can't buy, is it?'

'That's all I have at the moment,' I said, indicating the notes.

Harry picked it up. 'No problem, we can settle up next time,' he said, smiling. 'How did it go anyway, Martin?'

'How did what go?' I asked.

'How did the concert go? Your mum said you had a band over from Dublin at the house, and they were giving a concert, traditional Irish music, lovely. Your mum said the chocolate biscuits were for the interval. So how did the concert go?'

I think my mouth fell open somewhere about now. I sighed. I was getting good at sighing.

'The concert was great, thanks Harry,' I replied, and walked out.

Outside the shop I called Andrew. He laughed that much I thought he was going to wet his pants.

'Come on down anyway,' he said, 'I'll buy you a pint.'

I sat with Andrew that afternoon, we had a few beers, we talked and laughed. It did me the world of good. I loved my mum, and I felt privileged in a way to look after her, but it was very physically and mentally draining. It's a hard thing to admit, but sometimes I just needed to get away from her. I needed to be able to relax, and to talk to someone who lived in the same world that I did. I don't suppose for a moment Andrew knew how grateful I was for his company, and we would have both been embarrassed if I had told him, but I guess that's what mates are for.

* * * * *

As we sat and sipped, my mobile phone rang. It was Wendy, my ex-wife.

'Hi,' she said. 'Your mum's just turned up here... She's lost and confused. Can you come and collect her? Quick as you can, because we're all supposed to be going out.'

I sighed. I shook hands with Andrew, explained the situation, thanked him for his generosity, and left.

A few minutes later my mobile rang a second time. It was Wendy again.

'Hi, are you coming? We're waiting to go out!'

'Yes, I'm coming. I haven't got the car, I'm walking down,' I said.

'Well, quick as you can then.'

The line went dead.

The unseen tentacles of Alzheimer's reach out in all directions at once, spreading like the underground roots of a great tree, entwining themselves in every aspect of dozens of lives. No family member can be left untouched; here they had cut short my one afternoon in the pub, even when my mother wasn't there, and were affecting my ex-wife and our children.

I knocked on the door of the house where I had once lived.

'Hi,' said Wendy, opening it. She had her coat on. 'Sorry about rushing you like this, but we have to get into town. She just turned up a few minutes ago.'

'No problem,' I said, as I moved past her and into the lounge.

Rebecca and Daniel, my children, were standing with their coats on.

'Hi dad,' they said together.

'Hi both,' I replied. 'Sorry this is such a short visit, but I know you're trying to get out.'

Daniel shrugged his shoulders, 'No worries,' he said, with a big grin on his face.

'Come on, mum,' I said, 'we have to get you home.'

'I haven't finished my tea yet,' replied mum, putting down the cup and saucer.

'I'll make you another cup when we get home,' I replied. 'Wendy and Rebecca and Daniel are waiting to go into town.'

'Well, I'm not stopping them!' replied mum.

I held her coat for her: she put her arm into the wrong sleeve.

'Are we all going into town together?' she asked, trying to pull the other arm into the pocket instead of the sleeve, failing and trying again by moving around in a circle, like a dog chasing its tail. She failed again and moved around a bit more. We started to move around in circles together. Wendy began to sigh about then, I think. Rebecca looked at the ceiling and Daniel started to laugh.

'Come here,' said Wendy trying to help, and then the kids joined in. The five of us were all moving around in a slow, unwieldy circle as mum, in the middle of all this, thrashed about trying to get her coat on. Eventually the task was completed somehow and we moved out to the street.

Mum and I waved goodbye and began to walk home.

'You can't keep turning up there uninvited like this mum,' I said. 'That's the fourth time this week.'

'So what?' she said, indignantly. 'It's my house.'

'It isn't your house!' I exclaimed. 'It's Wendy's house, and you don't live there.'

'I *used* to live there,' she said.

'You've never lived there! Wendy and your grandchildren live there.'

'Where do I live, then?' said mum.

This is where I began to sigh again.

'You live with me at your own house.'

She seemed to be reflecting on this as we walked along. After a few minutes of uninterrupted silence, she suddenly asked: 'What does it look like?'

By then I had forgotten what we had been talking about.

'What does what look like?' I replied, puzzled.

'My house.'

Our conversations were often like this. I thought again about what the consultant had said back in 2002, about the rug of her memories being rolled up. That consultation seemed like a lifetime ago now. It struck me that a lot of what we are, and who we are, is the fabric of memories we carry around with us. Knowledge of our past roots us in our present, giving us focus in the current moment. When that knowledge becomes distorted or confused our roots wither, and our understanding of our own selves becomes destabilised. When that happens all the cushions disappear, and the world must seem a very harsh and uncertain place indeed.

'It's a lovely house,' I replied, 'it's where the Irish band plays, and the little girl in the radiator lives, remember?'

41

'Ah yes, I remember now,' said mum. 'But that's not my house.'

'Yes it is.'

'I don't remember ever buying that house.'

'You bought it with dad, years ago.'

We walked on again in silence for a while.

A policeman and policewoman were walking slowly towards us. When the four of us were just about to pass mum spoke to the policewoman.

'Hello!' said mum, as though she had known the officer all her life. 'Is your mother better now?'

The policewoman looked at mum, obviously trying to recall who she was.

'I must tell you this story about me and your mum,' continued my mother. 'One day when Benny and Frank had gone out for a drink, your mum and me were looking after Richard. He was very naughty when he was small, wasn't he?'

The policewoman looked at me.

'She has Alzheimer's,' I said, softly.

The two officers nodded.

'Anyway,' resumed mum, 'Richard wasn't let out because he was so naughty, and me and your mother...'

The story went on and on for at least the next 15 minutes. The two police officers paid attention to mum, and smiled and nodded in all the right places. I liked them both for that. As mum pressed on with her story, the policeman moved around to my side.

'Is she all right?' he whispered.

'She's my mum,' I replied quietly. 'She's been diagnosed with Alzheimer's disease. Do you know what that is?'

He nodded. 'I've seen it before. My grandfather thought there was a lake in his bedroom, he used to go fishing up there.'

The officer said this so matter-of-factly that I began to wonder just how widespread Alzheimer's was amongst the elderly population. I began to do some basic research after that, and the findings left me dumbstruck.

'Well, we must be going, now,' said mum. 'Give my love to your mother.'

'I will,' replied the policewoman, smiling.

'Her mother was very funny,' said mum as we walked on down the street.

I wondered: had she known the woman? She'd certainly spoken of her with firm conviction, and it was infectious. I doubted it, but I wasn't sure. Any onlooker would certainly have believed that the two women really were old friends.

'You told the little girl in the radiator I said she could come out, didn't you?' I asked, after a while.

'Yes, I did,' replied mum, nodding her head with conviction.

'What did she say?'

Mum shook her head. 'She said it isn't as easy as that.'

5. Our Last Christmas Dinner

WHEN MUM HAD gone to bed on Christmas Eve, I ventured out into the back garden to take a look at Godzilla the Goose. I checked its flesh for small bites and claw marks: there were none. I lifted it up and smelled it; as far as I could tell, the meat had not gone off.

I admit I had terrible misgivings about cooking the thing after it had been sitting in the garden all that time, but what with one thing and another I hadn't got around to replacing it with a normal turkey so it was Godzilla or nothing. I dragged it off the garden chair, and carried it over my shoulder, like a wounded soldier, back into the house. It needed to be washed thoroughly, and as it was too big to fit into the kitchen sink I gave it a bath. It lay there like a well-behaved child as I washed it down and dried it with a towel. Then I dragged it back into the kitchen. I had searched the internet for a good recipe for cooking goose, and had managed to find a tray large enough for the damn thing to lie on. For the next hour or so I prepared the monster for a very slow overnight cook. I would roast it raised on a drip tray; underneath I would put potatoes, carrots and parsnips, which would baste in the dripping fat.

This seemed like a splendid plan, until I raised the prepared carcass up to the oven and realised it wouldn't go through the door.

'Oh, bollocks!'

I slammed the giant bird back down onto the kitchen table. In a temper I went to get dad's saw from the garage. There wasn't too much rust on the blade, I thought, so I began the bloody dismemberment of mum's monster goose.

'Why the hell couldn't she just buy a normal turkey like anybody else?' I said to myself as I hacked through bone and sinew, tossing the discarded pieces, one after the other into the pan.

At last it was dissected into around six pieces, and I put the whole contraption into the oven on a low heat. I had a few presents to wrap, and to place under the Christmas tree before I fell into bed, exhausted.

The next morning at breakfast, mum asked me the same question she had asked me every day for the past month.

'Is it Christmas yet?'

'Yes, it is!' I said. 'Happy Christmas, mum.'

She gave a girlish squeal of delight and clapped her hands.

'Can we open our presents now?' she said.

We went to the tree. She unwrapped a woollen cardigan I had bought her. She put it on and kissed me.

'It's beautiful,' she said. 'Thank you very much.'

I gave her a gift from Peggy. Her sister had been dead for five years, but mum still talked to her all the time so I reasoned that the least she could do was buy mum a Christmas present. It was a leather handbag I had seen in town.

'Oh, she shouldn't have spent so much money,' said mum, 'but Peggy always did give lovely presents.'

'Aunt Peggy will be glad you like it,' I said.

'What have you got?' asked mum. 'I didn't buy any presents. I'm sorry.'

She looked very sad, and embarrassed. Unfortunately, it wasn't safe to allow her out on her own, so she hadn't had any opportunity to get me anything; I'd known she would become angry with herself over this, thinking that she had forgotten, and that that would have made her even more upset and confused.

'Yes, you did,' I said. 'This one's to me, from you.'

I carefully unwrapped a pair of my old trousers which I had taken out of my wardrobe and wrapped up for myself the previous night.

'Gee, thanks mum,' I said, and kissed her. 'They're great!'

'I hope you like them,' said mum. 'I hope they fit.'

'Sure they will,' I replied, and, being as I'd been wearing them only two days earlier, it was a pretty safe bet.

I also knew by then that Alzheimer's has a funny way of filling up the blanks in a sufferer's memory. I only had to act as though the present was from her to me, to let her see me unwrap it, and her mind would colour in the missing memory of her buying it for me.

'It took me a long time to find those trousers for you,' she said. 'The man in the shop said they were a very good quality pair.'

'Yes, they are, mum,' I said. 'Thanks a lot.'

I also had a nice shirt from her. Mum was happy; she hadn't forgotten her Christmas shopping, after all.

'Why don't you go and watch the telly, and I'll check on the dinner?' I said.

The dismembered goose seemed to be doing fine. Its sojourn in the garden didn't seem to have had a detrimental effect on the meat at all, and neither had its being carved up with a rusty saw. For all of the unconventionality of that Christmas, our last one together, it was going to be okay.

The smell of roast goose filled the little bungalow, and mum asked if she could lay out the table.

'That's a good idea,' I replied.

We didn't have a dining room, and our kitchen table would only seat four people. Mum shook her head, firmly; that wouldn't be big enough, she said. So she started to lay out places all around the house. Knives, forks and spoons were placed on the television, on top of each radiator, on the kitchen worktops, on the seat of each armchair – in fact, on any flat and level surface in the house that was more than a few inches wide. It seemed the Irish band and the little girl in the radiator would be joining us, too.

'You can't leave people out when they're in the house,' whispered mum. 'That would be so *rude*.'

'Is the little girl in the radiator going to come out to eat her dinner, then?' I asked, wondering how she would handle that one.

'She might be able to,' replied mum, 'but she'll have to go back in as soon as she's had her meal.'

'I thought she couldn't get out?' I said.

Mum thought for a moment. 'No, she can't,' she said. 'I suppose she'll just have to eat her dinner in there.'

I busied myself with the rest of the paraphernalia which traditionally goes with Christmas dinner, and mum watched television. At the back of my mind I was still worried about the recent history of the goose, and the possibility of food poisoning – especially since I was supposed to be looking after her – but it was too late to abandon it all and go out to a restaurant instead. Then I had an idea. For years, a ginger cat who lived locally had come into our back garden to play and hide in the bushes. He visited my parent's bungalow at least twice a week, and my dad had made a pal of him by giving him fresh fish on a Friday – my parents being traditional Catholics, they usually ate fish on Fridays. The old tom was in the garden right now, as luck would have it. I cut a nice slice of the hot goose flesh and carried it to the back door. The cat saw me immediately. I threw the meat to a spot about a foot in front of where he was sitting.

If the meat was poisoned, surely the cat would know it, and not eat it? If he rejected the goose, I reasoned, so would we. The cat sniffed the air, and cautiously moved forwards. I watched with baited breath as he sniffed the meat again, and then started to eat it. Once he was done, he stood up, now very alert, and licked his lips; I think I licked mine. I threw him another piece (we had plenty to spare), and he pounced on it straight away. I felt easier in my mind, then – though, fleetingly, I wondered whether I should really be placing all of my trust in him. What if he wasn't as smart as I was giving him credit for? Then we'd all be ill. I dismissed these worries with the same reckless attitude with which an alcoholic ignores a final demand letter from his landlord. *It'll be all right*, I thought, and set about the goose. It was time to dish up.

Mum insisted our 'guests' were well fed, and went around the house putting healthy amounts of goose on each plate. When she was finished there were a few slices and a leg each for ourselves: they were so big they looked like they had belonged to a professional sprinter. Then we sat down to that little kitchen table and quietly ate our last Christmas dinner together, she in her own little world and me in mine. We were two people in a bubble which excluded the rest of humanity; and within that was another bubble which contained only my mother. Alzheimer's is the ultimate isolation, the last and greatest loneliness. There we sat, the invalid and the carer, the prisoner and the jailer. She was blithely unaware of these thoughts, which were perhaps slightly maudlin; in fact, I couldn't remember seeing her so happy since my father had died.

As we ate, I pondered; I'd had a chat with Mary next door earlier in the week. She'd been adamant that it was time to think about finding a home for mum; maybe she was right? I was certainly struggling to cope on my own. I was an only child, with no brothers or sisters to share the load and the responsibility; my surviving aunts and uncles all lived in Ireland. There was no-one else.

I hated the idea of packing her off, and put it to the back of my mind.

'This turkey is lovely,' observed mum, breaking the silence, 'but it's a bit more greasy than usual.'

Probably because it's a goose, I thought.

'Peggy never ate enough green vegetables,' said mum. 'Me mammy is always telling her. Did you know there's iron in vegetables?'

'No, I didn't know that, mum.'

'Me mammy told me that only yesterday.'

My grandmother died 40 years ago.

'Me mammy said, *You'll always be healthy, Rose, if you eat your green vegetables.*'

There was a brief silence, during which I digested this.

Then mum spoke again. 'Did I ever tell you that there's iron in green vegetables?'

'No, I never heard that before.'

'Me mammy told me that.'

'Does the little girl in the radiator like her dinner?' I asked, changing the subject; the conversation was likely to go around and around in circles, otherwise, with me being told that there was iron in vegetables over and over again for the rest of the afternoon.

(A few weeks previously, mum had told me a joke, and had laughed as she told the story. A few minutes later she had forgotten that she had just told me the joke and so she told it to me again. Because she had forgotten she had previously said it, it was just as funny to her the second time. A few minutes later she had forgotten she had just told it twice, and so she told me the same joke, word for word again, and again she had laughed all the way to the punchline because she had forgotten she had already said it twice. Each time she told it, only a few minutes apart, it was as fresh and as funny to her as it had been the first time. The effect on the listener is, of course, somewhat different. The first time you laugh because it's a funny joke; the second time you laugh because they laugh, and that's infectious. The third time you laugh because the situation is so mad. The fourth time it starts to get scary. By the tenth time you want to leap out of the window to get away.)

'She says it's the nicest Christmas dinner she's ever had,' replied mum.

We served the traditional plum duff pudding after the meal, giving smallish portions to the band and the little girl in the radiator.

'They all said they didn't want a large helping, mum,' I said.

After dinner we cleaned all nine of the plates away from around the house and washed up. I went to turn the telly on – there was some film or other on I'd thought we could watch – but mum held up a hand.

'The band are going to play a few tunes for us,' she said.

So I sat back down, and watched while she moved her leg in time to the music in her mind, smiling and remembering and nodding her head all the way through the recital. Perhaps the songs she was listening to were those she and my dad had danced to all those years ago in Dublin – I remembered him telling me how he and mum had first met at a dance hall in the city. There was certainly a rare bliss on my mother's face that Christmas afternoon, as Michael and the rest of his imaginary band transported her back five decades to another time and another place – to a polished parquet dance floor, and she was a young girl again, with all of her life stretching out before her like an uncharted ocean.

I wondered how a healthy mind and spirit could ever come to this.

6. Bruno's Bare Bum

THREE OR FOUR MONTHS earlier, I had joined an internet dating site. It gave me something to do in the evening, and offered the chance to talk to some 'normal' women now and then. I'd been out on a few dates, and on the whole they had gone well. One night, one of the ladies had even come to dinner.

'What's the weather like in Germany, Anna?' mum had asked suddenly as we ate.

Anna and I looked at each other, both slightly perplexed by the question, though I had briefed her before she came into the house.

'I don't know, Rose,' said Anna.

'Well, how long have you been over here?' asked mum.

'Erm... I *live* here,' said Anna. 'I mean, I only live a few miles away.'

'You've picked up the language really quickly,' observed mum, 'and you seem to have lost your accent.'

'Anna's not German, mum,' I explained. 'She's from Rugby.'

'A German parachutist came down in Dublin once,' said mum, oblivious. 'During the war. He landed in Bath Avenue. It was all over the papers. Did you know him?'

'Anna's too young to have been in the war,' I said. 'And she isn't German, anyway.'

Mum pondered this for a bit. 'I'd have thought you would have been a bit more blonde,' she said, eventually.

I won't recite the rest of the dinner conversation here; suffice it to say that there was no shifting from mum's head the idea that my dinner date was German. I never saw Anna again.

I had made quite a few friends on the site, and one of them – Marianne – was having to leave her home and move into a flat. She didn't go into too much detail, but I got the impression that money was scarce and she was desperate. She seemed nice enough, and when she told me how she was going to have to have her dog put down, as the new landlord had specified there were to be no pets under any circumstances, my heart went out to her. I asked her why she didn't give the dog to the RSPCA; she said that 'Bruno' was not good with strangers, and had frightened the people at the local shelter. She assured me that he was the kindest, most loving dog anyone could ever hope to have, and, in a moment of foolish weakness, I agreed to take him in for a few weeks until Marianne got herself back on her feet. Bruno was in a kennel about a hundred miles south of where I lived, and I arranged with the kennel owner to drive down on the Saturday morning and take him home with me.

I've always loved animals, and they have always seemed to like me, too. So I didn't really think twice about giving Bruno a home for a short while. I thought it might give mum an interest, and perhaps take her mind off her fantasies for a while. He would also give her some responsibility during the day while I was at work, and would deter anyone from trying to force their way into the house. From a lot of angles, it seemed like having a dog to stay for a while was a very good idea.

I told mum about Bruno and she seemed thrilled. She'd had a little poodle called Sandy years ago, and had cried when he had eventually died of old age.

'It will be great to have a dog about the house again,' she declared.

So when Saturday morning came around, I kissed mum, locked her into the house, said I wouldn't be long, and set off to fetch Bruno.

It took me around two hours to get to the village. The drive down was pleasant, winding through countryside, the sight of green fields and hedgerows enlivening my spirits. The kennel was situated next to a farm; I found it, pulled through the gate and stopped. It was a dilapidated old place, with rusty sheets of corrugated iron thrown here and there against walls and chickens wandering about. An old lady's head wrapped in a red scarf emerged from around an open door. She seemed to be struggling with something heavy inside the red brick outbuilding.

'I've come for Bruno,' I announced cheerily.

'And you can bloody well have 'im!' she shouted back, and her head disappeared inside again.

She reappeared momentarily, heaving herself through the door and dragging one leg behind her as she walked. At first, I wondered if she was disabled; but then I saw that she had to walk like that because a medium-sized brown dog was attached to her right leg. It was clutching her waist with its forelegs and pumping its rear at her thigh, growling fiercely and showing a row of snow-white, sharp teeth the whole time. As the old woman moved down the path, the dog was hopping on its back legs to keep up with her.

'He does this sometimes,' she shouted at me breathlessly, as she laboured down the path towards me. The dog was still pumping away and growling the whole time. 'It's best to leave him to it. He'll be finished in a minute.'

Sure enough, at that the dog stopped growling and let go, dropping down to all fours and looking quizzically up at me. He was out of breath, and started to pant; his tongue was hanging out of his mouth, and a long line of saliva dribbled its way down to the ground. The old woman picked up the loose end of a rope which had been trailing along the floor. The other end was knotted around the dog's neck.

'Told you he wouldn't be long,' she said.

Bruno was the strangest looking dog I have ever seen. There was definitely some Alsatian in him, especially the coat and tail, and a bit of terrier, but the rest of the breeds mixed into him were unfathomable. His snout was long and thin like a Doberman's, and he had huge feet like a Great Dane's. His ears stuck out horizontally, like Yoda's.

'What sort is he?' I asked.

'Fuck knows!' she gasped. 'Here, take him.'

The old woman handed Bruno over to me, and immediately he began to snarl and show me his fine, long, white teeth.

'Careful!' warned the old woman, retreating back into the barn. 'He bites.'

I took one end of the old rope very carefully; Bruno pulled away from me on the other, snarling all the time.

'Hello, Bruno!' I said, in as cheery and friendly a way as I could. I remembered that everyone says a dog can tell when you're scared. 'Who's a good boy, then!'

Immediately, he charged forwards and leapt into the air, his front paws smacking me squarely in the middle of the chest; then, in one smooth movement, he pushed himself off me and then hit the ground running. Clearly, he thought he was making a bolt for it.

'Jesus!' I shouted. I hadn't expected that, and my heart started to thump madly in my chest. Somehow I managed to keep hold of the rope.

After gaining some measure of composure, I decided to take Bruno for a walk so we might get to know one another. Maybe familiarity with me might calm him down a bit.

'Come on, Bruno,' I said, and we set off down the farm track, back to the road.

He began to walk on the rope fairly well, but every second or two he would give me a suspicious glance, and I knew he was as wary of me as I was of him. We headed down the track, along the road for a bit and then back into the farm by a second rutted driveway. By the time we were back where we'd started, after a few hundred yards or so, the dog seemed to be lightening up a bit.

'Good boy, Bruno,' I said, and we stopped.

He looked at me, and I looked at him. I didn't really know what to do next. I decided to talk to him. I knelt down in front of him, so I wouldn't be towering over him, and might not look quite so intimidating.

'Are we going to be friends?' I said.

Bruno bared his teeth, but didn't growl. I had brought with me some dog chews, and I brought one out of my pocket, and waved it gingerly in front of his face.

'Do you want this?' I asked.

Bruno licked his lips.

'Are you going to be a good boy?' I asked.

He licked his lips again. Very slowly and carefully, I reached forwards with the chew, and Bruno took it gently from me. When it was in his mouth I seized the opportunity to stroke him. It would have been hard for him to bite me with a great big dog chew already in his jaws.

'Good boy, Bruno,' I said, stroking his head. 'Let's go round again!'

We set off down the track once more. This time he didn't pull on the rope, and didn't seem to glance so suspiciously at me as we went. When we completed the second circuit, I gave him another chew.

'Once more round, I think,' I said, and we set off again.

This time Bruno walked beside me, and didn't warn me when I petted him. He seemed to understand that I meant him no harm; I hoped he was started to feel similarly benign towards me. And when we completed the third circuit of the farm, Bruno seemed a much happier dog.

'Time to get into the car, and take you home, mate,' I said.

I opened the rear car door and Bruno jumped straight in. He was obviously used to travelling in a car. He sat in the rear passenger seat, like a person might, and I started the engine and drove down the farm track to the road.

We hadn't been going for more than a couple of minutes when it started. Bruno leaned forwards and, with his mouth about an inch and a half from my left ear, started to growl. I was in traffic by this time, and couldn't pull over. I began to sweat: I really thought he was going to bite me in the back of my head.

'There's a good boy!' I shouted as we sped along. 'Who's a good boy, then?'

Bruno continued to growl deep and low, the sort of growl that comes from deep in a dog's chest. He growled continuously as we went along. It was the most unnerving experience of my life. The more I tried to reassure him, the deeper and louder he growled, and the whole time his mouth was never more than two inches away from my left ear. He was so close to my head that I could feel his warm breath on the side of my neck the entire way home.

Two and a half hours later I pulled into mum's drive with a blinding headache, and Bruno still growling in my left ear.

I opened my door and got out. My shirt was wringing wet with sweat all down my back. I opened the rear door, took hold of his rope and pulled gently.

'Come on boy,' I said. 'Let's go inside.'

He refused to budge. I pulled harder on his rope, but he wouldn't move off the back seat. Finally, in an effort to show him that he was going to have to behave I shouted at him. 'Bruno!' I bawled. 'Get out of the fucking car!'

He jumped out. I wondered what his home life had been like before. I opened the front door and led Bruno into the house. In case he was unfriendly with mum, I decided not to let go of his rope until he and she had become acquainted.

'Mum,' I called as we came into the kitchen, 'this is Bruno.'

Bruno ran around mum's legs, sniffing her.

Mum handed Bruno a cheese sandwich which he took from her straight away.

'Hello, Barney,' she said. 'I made you some supper.'

Bruno sat in the kitchen with the cheese sandwich in his mouth, looking at mum. When mum moved into the front room, Bruno followed her. When she sat in the armchair, Bruno climbed up beside her on the seat, the cheese sandwich still in his mouth.

'Get down,' said mum, and Bruno got down.

Mum took the cheese sandwich from Bruno, he chewed what was left in his mouth, and mum reached over, opened his mouth and popped in a whole tomato.

'Good boy, Boris,' she said.

I had never seen a dog register true surprise on its face before, but when Bruno felt the whole tomato on his tongue it must have been a new sensation for him. He looked both surprised and bewildered. His eyes opened wide and he looked at me.

That was the beginning of an extraordinary friendship between my mother and this strange dog. Bruno ate what we ate. I came home from work one day to see him eating beans on toast, followed by chocolate biscuits. He had a wonderful way of dealing with baked beans on toast. Somehow, he would manage to lift the slice of toast still intact, very carefully out of his bowl, with the beans dripping off the end of it; then when he had raised the slice high enough into the air, he would shake his head as violently from side to side as he possibly could. I used to really hate the sound of the beans splattering up the front of the fridge, up mum's legs, up the wallpaper, and up my clothes from hem to hat.

He often had cheese sandwiches, and he seemed to like the odd battered fish. A full English breakfast was always his favourite, though: bacon, sausage, fried egg, beans, hash brown, mushrooms, tomatoes, black pudding and toast. He had a cup of tea with the band in the afternoon, said mum, and on Fridays they all had cream cakes: mum, the Irish band, the little girl in the radiator, and Bruno. Cold custard slices and jam doughnuts were his favourites, she said.

I knew nothing about Bruno's history, but I got the impression he had not been that well treated. As I watched them cuddling together in the armchair one evening, it struck me that they were both lost souls in what could be a very confusing and often painful world, and for the short time Bruno was with us each had found a soul mate, a companion to cling to when the world became mysterious and unpredictable.

One evening, when Bruno had been with us a couple of weeks, I came home from work and looked at him. Have you ever seen something so unexpected and strange that you just can't take your eyes off it? You keep staring at it, because you really can't believe the evidence of your own senses?

Bruno was in the conservatory and I was watching him through the kitchen window. I kept looking at him, trying to understand what I was seeing. When he turned sideways I saw the full picture. I think my mouth dropped open. From the top of his hind legs to the base of his tail, all his hair had gone. He had a completely pink bottom. I continued to stare in disbelief.

'What's happened to Bruno's backside?' I asked mum, unable to take my eyes off the dog's rear.

'I don't know,' said mum.

'What do you mean, you don't know?' I asked. 'He's got no hair on his backside!'

'Ask Peggy!' replied mum, defensively. 'Maybe she did it.'

I went out into the conservatory. Bruno was pleased to see me. I knelt down in front of him and ran my hand down his flank. His backside had been shaved as clean as a whistle, right down to the skin. Bruno licked my face and skipped about. When mum came out to the conservatory Bruno immediately sat down and looked at her warily. He wasn't about to go through that again, was the obvious message.

Mum shook her head. 'Isn't Peggy a bitch for doing that?' she said.

In the bin in the bathroom I found one of my disposable razors, several tissues, and piles of Bruno's hair. It was all so bizarre I didn't know what to say.

I thought about the intimidating and snarling canine Bruno had been when I first met him a few short weeks previously. Here was the hound the old lady had been pleased to see the back of. Here was the fierce guard dog who had tried to eat the postman and the paper boy every morning. Yet he must have stood calmly by and let my mother shave all the hair off his backside.

'Why did you do that, mum?' I asked. 'What for?'

'I didn't do anything!' she replied. 'What are you asking me for?'

It was pointless to try and get to the bottom of it, if you'll excuse the pun. Mum would only have got confused and upset. It was best to try and ignore it, if that were possible.

We now lived in a house festooned with dozens of my socks hung from every ceiling and wall, with a Christmas tree in the lounge – by now, it was almost spring – an invisible six piece Irish band, a little girl trapped inside the heating system, and a dog with a shaved backside.

Normality is a subjective concept.

I was chatting one night with Bruno's owner on the internet, and she asked me how he was getting on. I emailed her a picture of Bruno and my mother sitting together in the armchair. I carefully cropped the photograph so Bruno was only showing from the chest up, and told her he was doing fine.

Towards the end of January I met a new friend on the dating site. Her name was Heather and coincidentally she lived only a few miles from me in Coventry. We had gone to a local curry house for our first date, the first week in February, and I had told her about mum. She didn't seem fazed about it at all, and said she would love to meet her. I took the decision to tell mum about Heather.

'Mum,' I said casually, one evening. 'I've got a new girlfriend, and her name's Heather.'

'You can't do that!' she said, shocked. 'You're married to Wendy.'

'I've told you,' I said. 'We're getting divorced.'

'Who is?'

'Me and Wendy.'

'Have you told Wendy that?'

It was probably about this point where I started to sigh again.

'Of course, I've told her. She told me! I've moved out. I'm living here with you, aren't I?'

'Well, I don't know!' said mum. 'Nobody tells me anything!'

'You don't know whether I'm living here or not?' I said.

Mum shook her head. 'No-one told me.'

'Mum, it's only a two-bedroomed bungalow, how could you not know I was living here?' I asked.

'Peggy should have told me, shouldn't she?' observed mum.

I ignored that one. 'What did you think I've been doing here for the past three months?'

'I don't know!' said mum, she was getting irritated. 'There's so many people in here, sometimes it gets so confusing. All this coming and going.'

'There's only the two of us,' I said.

Mum smiled at me as though I was having a joke. 'Now, you *know* that's not true,' she said.

I decided to steer the conversation back to its original point. 'Heather's going to come round one evening,' I said. 'She'd like to meet you.'

'Well, bring her around, then,' said mum. 'We'll just have to find some room for her, from somewhere.' And then, as an afterthought, 'Does she like chocolate biscuits?'

7. Bruno Settles In

BRUNO SOON CAME to think of the bungalow as his own personal kennel. He was in many ways a wonderful dog, and he did mum a world of good just by being around, but there were a few times when I wondered if his real owner had been entirely honest about him.

He would do what he was told if he happened to feel like it at the time; if he didn't, then he either pretended to be stone deaf, which was entirely implausible given the size of his ears, or he would just begin that awful deep growling, and bare his teeth.

'I think I'm going to enrol Bruno in some obedience classes, mum,' I said, one evening after supper.

'That's a great idea!' agreed mum. 'Can I take him?'

I felt the icy, cold warning of catastrophe flood over me like a wave. Mum and Bruno out together for the evening would end in disaster for sure. There would be a lawsuit at the very least.

'We'll all go together,' I said, trying to keep the sound of rising panic out of my voice.

I scanned the local papers, and found a class which met every Tuesday evening at a junior school gym not too far away. I rang the number.

'Oh, Mr Bruno sounds *too* delightful,' cooed a soft and melodious female voice, when I had explained why I was calling. 'Do bring him along on Tuesday… You never know, he might even meet some lovely lady doggies here.'

I tried to explain to the woman that I thought Bruno had some real behavioural problems, and that she should be prepared for what he was like.

'Please do not distress yourself, Mr Slevin,' she assured me. 'We have been dealing with gentleman dogs and their rakish ways for some time now (giggle), and I can honestly say that we are always able to improve their social skills to a remarkable degree. After a few weeks with us, our students can be taken out to any event at all with the utmost confidence of their owners. Think of us as a finishing school for our doggie friends.'

A finishing school! She wasn't even listening to me. I agreed to be there next Tuesday, and put the phone down. I looked at Bruno. I could swear he was smiling at me.

'Oh, bless him!' said mum.

When Tuesday rolled around Bruno and mum sat in the back of the car. He didn't make a sound as we pulled away from the house, and simply looked casually out of the window, mum's arm around him. I began to relax.

'I don't think Benny needs these classes, anyway,' said mum, at length. 'He's very well-behaved really.'

'Well, it might be fun,' I said, 'and he might enjoy it.'

We drove through the school gates, and went in to the car park. A silver Mercedes had pulled in just before us, and we watched a middle-aged woman in a well-cut trouser suit get out. She went around to the front passenger door and opened it. Very gracefully, a snow-white standard poodle with a pink ribbon in its hair exited the car, with considerably more poise than most people can manage. The woman took a long pink lead from her jacket pocket and clipped it neatly to the poodle's matching pink collar. Together they walked towards the gymnasium building as though on the seafront at Cannes or the catwalk of some canine fashion show, probably in Hollywood. My heart sank.

'That's a beautiful dog, over there,' observed mum.

'Yes it is,' I agreed, 'but I'm beginning to wonder if this is really the right place for Bruno.'

'Of course it is,' said mum, defending the good name of her new best friend. 'Why wouldn't it be?'

A black Jaguar rolled into the car park, stopped and let out a beautiful golden retriever who looked like he had just won a rosette at Crufts.

Bruno was watching all the dogs arriving with great interest. We got out of the car, and I took Bruno's lead from mum.

'Let me hold him,' I said, trying to think of all eventualities.

The school gym was like every other school gym: a large, rectangular building with a wooden floor, and taped lines for volleyball, football and various other games marked out on it. Small goal nets stood empty at either end.

In a militarily straight line, about a dozen people queued with their dogs, all of whom were perfectly behaved – I wondered why they needed to come here. Besides the white poodle and the retriever, there was a little white lhasa apso – he looked like it had taken his owner a month to brush him to perfection, with not a single hair out of place – and a brindle Staffordshire bull terrier, who stood so proud it was obvious he was on show and he knew it. There were other breeds I didn't know, some I had never seen before, but all were immaculately groomed and turned out, and all equally beautifully behaved. Their owners were dressed up, too; I got the impression the entire class might be going out to a top restaurant afterwards.

I didn't think mum, Bruno and I would be invited. I was in a pair of old jeans and a t-shirt with a hole in the back, and a brush-stroke of dried paint on the front, mum was mum and Bruno, especially, was Bruno. His horizontal ears and indeterminate lineage drew a few quizzical stares down the noses of the lined-up owners. His overall look was not improved by the fact that the hair on his backside hadn't quite grown back yet.

At the head of the line was a middle-aged woman, with a blue rinse hairdo, tweed skirt, beige cardigan and brown sensible shoes; she was taking money, and marking everyone's name down into a register. She was leaning over a school desk writing in the book, and had her back to us. I decided we should let her know that Mr Bruno and we had arrived. As it turned out, Bruno had his own way of introducing himself. I walked forwards, with as much dignity as I could manage. I could feel them all watching me, and I was enormously relieved when Bruno trotted along very nicely beside me. He was going to behave himself, thank God.

As we got to a couple of feet from the woman taking the money, it happened. Such is the sudden nature of catastrophe that you can find yourself in the middle of a full-scale disaster before you even know it's happening. One minute the school gymnasium was like an elegant and beautiful ocean liner, sailing majestically through an azure sea with her bejewelled passengers sipping dry Martinis and making small talk with the Captain; the next, she was listing at an angle of 30 degrees to starboard, klaxons were going off and all the passengers were running along the deck, screaming.

With the speed of a striking cobra, Bruno leapt forwards and caught the woman around the waist with his forelegs. He pressed her down onto the desk with such violence her glasses flew off and skidded along the floor and began to pump his thighs. As he pumped, he let out an horrific, satanic growl which filled the hall.

There was immediate uproar. The poor woman gave out a sort of strangled squeal, and all the dogs started to bark at once. The owner of the white poodle picked him up into her arms, but the dog was either so startled or frightened that it urinated a great jet out of her arms. The owner tried to aim it away from the people and animals who surrounded her, but everyone got some. The Staffordshire bull terrier immediately started to fight with every other dog in the place, and the retriever got loose and ran out of the gym, with his frantic owner hobbling after him in her high heels.

I dashed forwards and got hold of Bruno by the collar. I was going to pull him off the traumatised woman, but his snarling reaction was so vicious that I had to let go. The whole time Bruno was still pumping madly on the poor woman's leg and growling so loudly and baring his teeth that it literally terrified everyone, human and canine alike.

'I'm so sorry about this!' I shouted. 'He does this sometimes... Don't worry, he won't be long!'

There was bedlam all around us. The noise in the gym was deafening. The owners were shouting and trying to control their pets. The dogs were all barking, yelping, fighting and running around in all directions. Bruno was still growling and pumping the lady's leg with such violence that she had been reduced to a rag doll. I was shouting at Bruno, and mum was just standing there, saying nothing, but casually observing the mayhem with the detached professionalism of a seasoned war reporter. She was the calmest person in the whole place.

Eventually, Bruno finished and dropped down to all fours. He stood there with his horizontal ears cocked sideways, panting, and seemingly surprised at the uproar all around him.

I grabbed his lead and hauled him away from the woman who had been pinned to the desk throughout the entire proceedings.

'I can't apologise enough!' I said.

The woman stood up, she was squinting at me, as her glasses were still lying on the floor. I saw the spectacles, only a few feet from me, and walked forwards to retrieve them, but Bruno saw them first and dived on them.

'Give me those!' I said to him, as sternly as I could.

Bruno had the delicate spectacles in his mouth, and whenever we played this game at home with a stick, a play-fight would ensue, and Bruno would fight me for the toy.

'Let go!' I said, gently taking hold of one lens. As soon as I did so, Bruno shook his head violently and the spectacles snapped in the middle.

The sound of the little crack made my stomach turn over.

'For fuck's sake, let go!' I bawled into Bruno's ear.

'Tut, tut, tut, tut,' said someone behind me. I ignored it.

Bruno opened his mouth gently, allowing me to retrieve the broken spectacles.

I held up the two broken pieces to the woman. She said nothing, but held up her hand to stop us approaching any further.

Around us the carnage was evident. The bull terrier had been dragged into a corner of the room away from all the other dogs, and was now being quiet. The beautifully brushed little lhasa apso looked like it had just fallen into a cement mixer, and the white poodle was still in her owner's arms. The owner herself had dark circles and lines around her eyes where her mascara had run; she looked like she had been crying.

The molested instructor was now standing up at the desk, trying to salvage what was left of her dignity. Her tights were in shreds, and hung from her legs in long streamers across the floor.

'I think we'll go,' I said to the woman.

She didn't reply.

'Come on, mum,' I said. 'Let's get out of here.'

I walked Bruno back towards the door, and he trotted along very nicely on his lead. The bastard. Then mum said the line that will go down in our family history. Shielded by the armour plate of her Alzheimer's, and blissfully unaware of the social situation we were in, mum raised her arm as we departed and called out, 'It was lovely to meet you all.' And then, as we exited the room, 'See you all next Tuesday!'

Once in the fresh air, I breathed a sigh of relief. We reached the car.

'Get in!' I said to Bruno, holding the rear door open for him.

'Well, that went very well, I thought,' said mum. 'I'm not sure what he learned, though.'

I didn't say anything. I just started the car and drove away, with the reckless determination of a get-away driver after a bank job. In the rear view mirror I could see mum and Bruno cuddling on the back seat. Mum leaned down and gave Bruno a great big, lingering kiss on the top of his head. When she had finished Bruno gently licked her nose. There was a love light passing between them.

'Oh bless him!' she cooed.

8. Escape From The Bungalow

MUM WAS UP, washed, dressed and ready to go. She had her raincoat on, headscarf, and gloves. Her big handbag hung from the crook of her left arm, and her bus pass was in her right hand.

'I'm off now!' she called back over her shoulder. 'See you later.'

She couldn't get out of the house because I had turned the deadbolt key, and then had hidden the key in my room.

'The door's locked!' she called from the hallway. 'I can't get out.'

I tried to ignore her.

'Martin, I can't get out!' she called again.

'It's a quarter past three in the morning!' I shouted, pulling the pillow over my head.

'I have an appointment at the hairdresser's!' she shouted back. 'I can't get out!'

'It's a quarter past *three* in the bloody *morning*, mum!' I shouted. 'The hairdresser's doesn't open for six hours. Go back to bed!'

I could hear her step lightly along the hall carpet, and then disappear into her own room. I fell back to sleep.

She was back, *Groundhog Day*-like, before long.

'I'll see you later!' she called from the front door.

I awoke again with a start, and looked at the clock with one eye. It was four o'clock. I could hear the handle being rattled.

'Martin, the door's locked, I can't get out!'

I threw the duvet back with a violent sweep of my arm and sprang out of bed. I had had enough of this.

The effects and symptoms of Alzheimer's disease are many and varied; people reading this who have to deal with the disease in a loved one may recognise some of the scenes described here, and others will have different stories to tell. However, there does seem to be one aspect of the disease which appears to affect most sufferers, and that is a loss of the perception of time. The very concept seems utterly to lose its meaning; a clock face appears only as an abstract pattern of numbers and lines, and any meaning or significance to the pattern is lost. The phrase, 'Three o'clock' may as well be an equation in quantum physics.

'Mum!' I said, exasperatedly, 'it's the middle of the bloody night. It's four o'clock in the morning, I have to be up for work at seven, so please… GO TO BED!'

I went back into my room and crashed back between the sheets, so tired I could hardly think straight.

'IF I'M LATE FOR MY HAIR APPOINTMENT SHE WON'T DO IT!' bawled mum at the top of her voice.

I opened my eyes. She had followed me into the bedroom.

I jumped out of bed again. Mum ran from my room and into hers, and I chased her there.

'Get into bed this minute!' I shouted.

I was pointing at the bed like some irate dad, scolding a naughty child.

'I will not!' shouted mum.

'Yes, you will!'

'I WILL *NOT*!' repeated mum, her voice rising to a scream.

'Fine!' I said. 'Bloody well stay there then, but I have to get some sleep!'

I went back into my room, and somehow sleep came to me again. I had just drifted off again when I felt a pushing against my shoulder, and awoke again to find mum sitting on the side of the bed.

'I don't want to live here any more,' she said simply. 'I want to go back to my own house.'

It took me a couple of seconds to focus on the bedside clock. It was now 5am.

'This *is* your house,' I sighed.

'No, I mean my *real* house,' insisted mum. 'I want to go back there now.'

'This *is* your real house,' I growled.

'No it isn't,' replied mum, defiantly shaking her head.

'YES IT *IS*!' I shouted.

'NO IT *ISN'T*!' shouted back mum. She was sitting on the edge of my bed, and we were shouting at one another. Alzheimer's makes everyone crazy.

'I mean my *own* house, the one with the green kitchen floor,' said mum, in a suddenly softer voice.

I tried to calm down and think. No, I didn't know what she meant.

'We've never lived in a house with a green kitchen floor,' I said. 'Will you *please* go back to bed? Please?'

'It has a beautiful kitchen,' she said. 'All the cupboards are in real wood, and the floor is green.'

I was trying to remember that it wasn't mum's fault. I was trying not to get angry with her, but I was so tired I could hardly focus on the conversation.

'Just go to bed, please, mum!'

'I'll go to bed in my own house. I don't like it here any more, there's too much shouting.'

'You're doing most of the shouting,' I said. 'We've never *had* a house with a green floor, this *is* your house, I need some sleep, so *please*… go to bed!'

Mum began to rummage through her handbag, lifting out all sorts of things: a pair of mismatched gloves, a small umbrella, a shoe, a dirty coffee mug, endless bits of crumpled papers. She spread them all out on the bed, and started to unfold the papers, checking them one by one, and then replacing them carefully back into the bag. Finally, she straightened one out and showed it to me.

'Look!' she said, shoving the paper at me.

I looked at it; it was a bank statement.

'What are you showing me that for?'

'It's my hairdressing appointment,' said mum, 'and you're going to make me late.'

'It's a bank statement, mum, and it's now five in the morning,' I sighed. 'Please, go to bed.'

Suddenly there was a massive crash on the bed as Bruno landed on it. He had his lead in his mouth and his tail was going nineteen to the dozen.

'Oh, for Christ's sake!' I whimpered, burying my head in the pillow.

Mum got up and left the room, and Bruno followed her. I could hear her moving up and down the hallway. Then there was silence. I must have fallen asleep again. I was awoken by another shout.

'I'm going to tell the police about you keeping me a prisoner!' yelled mum from the hallway, suddenly. 'Then they'll put you in jail!'

'GO TO BED!' I screamed.

At 7am my alarm went off, and I dragged myself upright. I dressed, and looked into mum's room. She wasn't there. I found her asleep in the living room chair, still dressed, still wearing her headscarf. Bruno, lying at her feet, looked up at me, but didn't move. I decided not to disturb her. I dressed quietly, had some coffee, and left the house for work.

* * * * *

How I managed to get through that day without falling asleep I shall never know. It seemed endless but, eventually, with my shift over, I headed home.

As soon as I pulled up outside the house, Mary next door came to her front door and waved me over, anxiously. Mary's drive and mum's were side by side, with a small, wooden fence separating them; the two front doors were actually at the sides of each property, and faced each other.

'Bruno's been barking for hours!' said Mary. 'I think there's something wrong. My phone's not working so I couldn't ring you.'

My heart pumping, visions of what I might find, I put my key into the door. I could hear the dog going berserk. As soon as I turned the handle he barged past me and then ran back into the hall; excited and skittish, he started to run around the small bungalow, in and out of each of the rooms, whining and barking.

'Mum?' I called, but there was no answer. I checked every room, including the garage and the garden shed, but she was gone. How she'd got out I wasn't sure, but got out she had. Bruno sat down and looked at me, as if to say, 'What shall we do now?'

'Is everything all right?' said Mary, from her front door.

I went back outside. 'Mum's gone!' I said.

'Oh dear,' replied Mary. 'Ring the police – tell them she's missing.'

'I will,' I said, and called the police. I gave them a description of mum, and what she had been wearing when I had last seen her. They said they would notify any cars in the area and keep a lookout for her, and took my mobile telephone number. They also advised me to call the hospital.

I rang the Walsgrave, Coventry's main hospital, and waited while they checked their admissions for that afternoon; no-one answering mum's description had been seen there. They did have a woman who seemed very confused and lost, and whom they thought might have a form of dementia, but she was Afro-Caribbean. I wondered how many people with dementia were lost in a middling-sized city like Coventry at any given moment; there were at least two today.

I rang Wendy, on the off-chance that mum had gone there again.

'Yes,' said Wendy. 'She was here for hours, but she's gone now, she said she was going back home.'

'You should have held on to her!' I said. 'You shouldn't have let her go!'

'I'm sorry, I didn't think. She seemed all right to us. She stayed for a while, then she said she had a hair appointment, and she left. I had no reason to keep her.'

I apologised; it wasn't Wendy's fault. In fact, it wasn't anyone's fault but mine. I must have forgotten to turn the deadlock key when I had left for work that morning. She could have left any time she liked.

I looked at Bruno, sitting in the hallway, watching me closely, his horizontal ears pricked, rigid with anticipation.

'I wonder if you could find her?' I said to him. He turned his head to an angle, so that one ear was higher than the other, like a motorcycle leaning into a bend. 'It's worth a go,' I said.

I put the lead on his collar, and we went out into the street.

By now it was around 5pm, and I let Bruno take the lead. He sniffed at the floor, turned this way, and then that way, and finally headed off down the road towards the shops. We passed Harry's, and I stuck my head around the door.

'Hi, Harry,' I called. 'Have you seen my mum today?'

'Yes, Martin. She was in here about an hour ago,' he called back.

That was good news: we were getting warmer.

'Do I owe you any money?' I asked.

'No. She bought some chocolate biscuits, but she had her own money with her,' replied Harry, 'Is everything all right?'

'She's gone missing,' I said. 'She's basically lost.'

'Do you want me to come with you?' asked Harry.

I was very grateful. No wonder Harry's little shop was so popular with everyone on the estate.

'That would be great, Harry. Thank you very much.'

He said something to his wife in Urdu, and she went behind the counter while Harry put his coat on. His two sons were stacking shelves at the back of the shop. Harry shouted to them, and they stopped what they were doing and put their coats on, too.

'They can help,' he said to me.

'Thanks very much, Harry,' I said.

The two lads smiled at me as they passed, and went out into the street, heading back towards the bungalow.

'If you just drive around the local streets, Harry,' I said, 'I'll take the dog through the park.'

'No problem,' said Harry, as he got into his car.

Within minutes we had a mini search party organised, with people going off in all directions from the little shop. The big supermarkets were killing Harry's little business, and when they finally finished him off – as they did a few years after this – they also destroyed a focal point in the local community, one of those landmarks that helped glue it together. There was more to Harry's than just a shop: it was a part of the living estate, of our small community, and it was dying. Harry wasn't going down without a fight, but it was a battle he was doomed to lose.

Our local park is not that big, but it is well-used by local dog walkers and children. There is a play area for young kids, with slides and swings, and a skate bowl made of concrete where older kids on bikes and skateboards practise their skills with their friends. There were some kids in the skate bowl, and we started our search by walking over to them.

'Hi, lads,' I called out to the small group. One of them came over. 'Has anyone seen an elderly lady in a white raincoat?'

'I seen someone like that,' he said. 'She went up that way.'

He pointed to the far end of the park. I looked the way he pointed but couldn't see mum in the distance.

'How long ago was this?' I asked.

'Not long,' he replied. 'I ain't got a watch.'

'Thanks anyway,' I said, and we started off again the way the lad had indicated.

Bruno pulled on the lead with his nose to the ground, like an old-fashioned police bloodhound, and as we went on I suddenly saw a figure way in the distance; a small figure in a light-coloured raincoat. I knew it was mum straight away.

'There she is!' I said, and I noticed that Bruno had stopped and was staring at the figure, too. Mum was walking towards the far end of the park, where there was a small gated exit, which would lead her out onto the main road. If she managed to get onto a bus, we would lose her completely.

I knelt down and stroked Bruno. 'Go see mum!' I said to him, pointing towards the distant figure, and let his lead go. Bruno took off like a missile, with his lead flying in the air behind him.

I began to run behind him, but I was quickly out of breath. Bruno was surprisingly powerful and quick, for his size, and he covered the distance between us and mum in less than 20 seconds. I stopped to take a breath, and when I looked up Bruno had already reached her and was barking and running around her in circles. The smile of relief was just forming on my lips, but it froze as I saw mum reach down and pick up Bruno's lead before, to my horror, the two of them continued to trot off in the same direction, Bruno walking calmly beside her towards the park exit.

71

'Oh no!' I said, gasping for breath. 'You stupid bloody dog! You're not supposed to…'

I shouted Bruno and whistled him. I could see Bruno stop, and look back at me. I whistled him again, and this time he started to pull on his lead in the other direction. He was so much more powerful than mum, I could see her stop, and stand still as Bruno tugged on the lead; her whole body jerked as Bruno repeatedly pulled on his lead. I could see him pulling her right over, but eventually she went with him and changed direction. They started back towards me. I began to run again.

I could see mum looking towards me, and I waved. She waved back, and let Bruno go. The dog came flying back towards me, and began to bark when he reached me again. He seemed to enjoy this game. I picked up his lead and we hurried forwards to where mum was. Eventually we all met in the middle of the park.

I was determined not to fight with her. 'Where have you been all day?' I said, breathlessly.

'I don't know,' replied mum. 'I've been looking for the hairdresser's, but they've moved the shop.'

I couldn't help but laugh.

'It's not funny!' said mum. 'I haven't had my hair done in weeks. You don't understand!'

'I'll take you tomorrow,' I said. 'Is that okay?'

'Yes,' she said, and we all began to walk back to the other end of the park.

'I have to call into Harry's,' I said. 'I have to tell him something.'

'Can we get some chocolate biscuits?' asked mum.

'As many as you like,' I replied, 'and a big bone for Bruno!'

9. A Trip To The Hairdresser

IN THAT STRANGE no-man's land between being half awake and half asleep, I could hear the familiar sound of the front door rattling. I started to slowly drift back into wakeful consciousness.

'Martin, the door's locked, I can't get out,' came mum's familiar voice from the hallway.

It was a quarter past four in the morning the day after our escapade in the park. I groaned and turned over.

'I have an appointment with the hairdresser, and the door's locked,' she called again.

I took a deep breath, and hugged the pillow even tighter.

'Martin, the door's locked. I can't get to the hairdresser's.'

'It's too early,' I said. 'Go back to bed. We're not going to the hairdresser until midday.'

'I can't get out!' called mum from the hallway.

'Go back to bed!' I groaned. 'I'll tell you when it's time.'

'You might forget.'

'I won't forget. Go back to bed,' I answered. I was wide awake by now.

'You might forget,' she said again.

'I won't forget!'

'How do you know you won't forget?' asked mum.

'*What*?' I asked. I couldn't believe I was actually having this conversation.

'How will you remember not to forget?'

'I WON'T BLOODY FORGET! GO BACK TO BED… *PLEASE*!'

Bruno landed on the bed with an almighty crash. The whole bed shook. He had his new bone in his mouth, and staggered towards me, growling. I had learned to identify his different growls, and this was a friendly, 'Look at my lovely new bone!' sort of growl.

'Bed, Bruno!' I shouted. 'And mum, you go to bed too!'

Bruno sprang off the bed. I could hear her go back along the hallway, muttering as she went. 'You might forget,' I heard her say as a parting shot.

I sighed and turned over.

Some time later, I opened my eyes to see mum sitting on the end of my bed. It was a quarter past five. She was dressed to go out again, in the same raincoat and scarf. When she saw me look at her she said, 'You might forget. I'll wait here, just in case.'

Some people seem to have endless amounts of patience. People who build models of the Eiffel Tower out of matchsticks, for instance, or anglers – it must take enormous patience to sit by a riverbank for hours on end, waiting for a passing fish to bite. I had never envied people like that until mum got Alzheimer's; then I realised I just wasn't made like those saintly souls. In fact, the fuse of my temper was getting shorter and shorter every passing day. Looking back now, I realise I was in as much trouble as mum was, only I couldn't see it. Early on we'd had some support from social services, but the social worker had long since stopped visiting us and there was no-one else for us to talk to. I wasn't aware of any carer support organisations at that time, and I seemed to spend every day and every night standing with my toes sticking out over a cliff edge. I wonder how much of a final push I would have needed to have gone over for good.

I threw the covers back, and got out of bed.

'Are we going now?' asked mum.

'I'm going to make some breakfast,' I replied, putting on my dressing gown. 'I'm not going to be allowed to go back to sleep, am I?'

'I just didn't want you to forget,' said mum.

'I know,' I said. It wasn't as though she could help being this way. 'Do you want some eggs?'

'Have we got time?' asked mum.

By the time my 7am alarm went off a couple of hours later, it seemed like I had been up for days. I telephoned work and told them I wasn't feeling very well and I wouldn't be in. I had been taking a lot of time off lately, and I was running out of excuses; I got the feeling that my employers, like me, were losing patience. If I lost my job, God knew what would happen to the pair of us.

Mum sat at the kitchen table with me, and ate a hearty breakfast, still in her raincoat and headscarf. She wanted to be ready to leave at a moment's notice, as soon as I said it was time to go.

I had told her that she had a hairdressing appointment at midday, but to be honest that was just to shut her up and get her back into bed. So I trawled through the local Yellow Pages until I found a local salon who could fit her in that morning. The appointment was made for 11 o'clock; with 15 minutes to go we set off.

The salon was one of those trendy modern ones, all black and stainless steel, and when we arrived one of the hairdressers – who were also all dressed in black – came over to us.

'Hello,' she said, with a smile. 'I'm Tracy. Can I help you?'

'We have an appointment for 11 o'clock,' I said. 'Mrs Slevin?'

Tracy looked in the book. 'Oh yes, that's fine. Can I take your coat and scarf, Mrs Slevin?' She hung mum's things on a steel hook. 'What can we do for you this morning, Mrs Slevin?'

'I'd like a perm, and some colour,' replied mum. 'Can Barbara do it? I always have Barbara.'

Tracy looked confused. 'We don't have a Barbara here,' she said.

Mum started to put her coat back on. I intervened quickly.

'Mum, Barbara said Tracy can do it for you,' I said.

'Oh, that's all right then,' agreed mum. 'As long as Barbara said it's all right.'

She took her coat off again.

'Who's Barbara?' whispered Tracy.

'I have no idea,' I replied truthfully. 'She gets a little confused sometimes, that's all.'

Tracy nodded conspiratorially. 'I understand,' she said.

'Come and sit over here, Mrs Slevin,' said Tracy, indicating a free seat by a basin.

'Thank you, Barbara,' said mum, following Tracy over to the station.

I picked up a magazine and started to read a three-month-old gossip column.

Tracy fussed about and mum was smiling broadly.

'Have you retired, Mrs Slevin?' asked Tracy.

'Call me Rose,' replied mum.

'Have you retired, Rose?' asked Tracy.

'No, I'm a first class seamstress,' replied mum, proudly. 'I make curtains for Princess Margaret.'

Tracy stopped what she was doing. 'Really?' she gasped.

'Oh yes,' went on mum. 'I haven't been working lately because I'm being kept in a strange house. When I escaped they sent the dog out after me.'

Tracy was motionless, so were the other girls in the salon. I thought it was funny. I didn't say anything and continued to read the magazine as though I hadn't heard any of this.

'All they give me to eat is chocolate biscuits, and they make me very confused with all the shouting, and the comings and goings. We have a band though, and they play for me some evenings. Has your house got a green floor in the kitchen, Barbara?'

'No… no, our kitchen floor is cream,' replied Tracy.

'That's not it, then,' said mum, shaking her head sadly.

Tracy stood there frozen to the spot with a brush in one hand and a comb in the other. 'Sorry…' she said.

I had to smile. It still amazes me how far off-kilter people are thrown when confronted by a person with dementia. They never seem to know how to proceed or what to say.

'And there's a little girl that's a prisoner in there too,' went on mum.

When mum started on the little girl in the radiator, I knew it was going to be a long, and involved conversation. I got up and walked over to mum and Tracy.

'How long will this take?' I asked.

'Oh, a couple of hours at least,' replied Tracy.

The Craftsman pub was directly across the road from the salon, and it had just opened its doors. I had watched several regulars troop in.

'I'll be back in a little while,' I said to Tracy.

Tracy didn't look very confident when she realised I was leaving.

'She'll be fine,' I said to her. 'They're just stories.'

Tracy nodded and smiled, but the smile wasn't that convincing.

'Mum, I have to go for a message,' I said. 'I'll be back in a little while.'

'Yes, that's fine,' said mum, 'I'm just telling Barbara all about Mr Jackson.'

I had never heard mum mention anyone by the name of Mr Jackson before, and had no idea who he might be.

'Yeah, okay,' I said.

I left the salon and headed across the road to the pub. It was a lovely, clear crisp morning, and a couple of pints in the morning sunshine would go down very well.

'Don't normally see you in here this early,' remarked the landlord, as I walked to the bar. 'No work today?'

'I'm off sick,' I replied.

'Yeah, you look sick,' he replied, smiling, as he placed a cold lager on the bar top for me. I paid him and carried it outside, where I could watch the salon across the road. I felt a bit guilty about sitting there drinking beer when I should have been at work, and I suppose if one of my bosses had driven by at that moment and seen me, I might have got into trouble, but I felt I needed it. When you care for an Alzheimer's patient, their fantasies and delusions spread into your life as well. I'm not saying you believe the tales; you don't, you often know them to be untrue. But they still invade your time. You have to deal with them in one way or another, and you end up living sort of half in the real world, and half in the patient's world of historical fantasy and distorted memory. Separating one from the other each day is extremely tiring, mentally, and sometimes, like now, I just had to steal some time for myself, no matter how I got hold of it.

'Morning chap,' said an elderly gent, as he sat down at my table. 'Lovely weather.'

'Morning,' I replied. 'Yes it is.'

My companion opened out his newspaper and began to read. Having gone as far as commenting on the improved condition of the weather, he obviously felt he didn't need to speak to me any more. I didn't mind. The lager was cold and crisp, and I sat there out at the front of the pub just enjoying the peace of the moment. I knew mum was having a nice time across the street in the hairdresser's, and all was right with the world.

I finished my pint after a little while, and, working on the principle that no bird ever flew on one wing, I went back into the bar for another. Glass replenished, I came back out and resumed my seat. My companion looked up from his paper, saw me and nodded. A man of few words, obviously.

I was about halfway down my second beer when my friend suddenly pointed across the street. 'Aye, aye,' he said, 'something's happening over there!'

I followed his gaze, just in time to see mum running up the road. Her head was covered in a bright blue plastic cap, with her hair sticking out of it in all directions, and behind her was flapping a matching, bright blue plastic cape. Behind her in dogged pursuit was Tracy, and the other girls from the salon, all in black and running after mum in single file. They looked like a line of crows moving over a field.

'Oh, hell!' I said, 'I'll be back in a minute.'

I left the pub car park, and raced across the road. Tracy and the gang had caught up with mum by the time I reached them.

'What's happened?' I asked.

'She just got up and ran out!' exclaimed Tracy.

'Come on, mum,' I said. 'The girls haven't finished doing your hair yet.'

'I saw somebody I knew,' explained mum. 'Somebody I used to go to school with.'

'Yeah, well, you can talk to her later,' I replied, 'but right now you have to go back with Tracy to have your hair finished.'

'Oh yes, of course,' agreed mum. 'Come on, Barbara.'

With that she led the little procession back to the salon.

When we all piled back into the hairdresser's Tracy was looking seriously concerned. 'Can you stay with her?' she said. 'In case she decides to run off again?'

'I'll tell you what,' I said, reaching around to my back pocket as though to retrieve something from them, 'take my handcuffs, and if she gives you any more trouble, just cuff her to the chair.'

Tracy's face was a picture. Her mouth fell open and she recoiled physically backwards in horror. 'We can't do that!' she gasped, 'she's a customer!'

'They always cuff her at the other place,' I said, innocently.

'Indeed they do,' agreed mum, helpfully.

I thought Tracy was going to cry.

'I'm only kidding,' I said.

Tracy and the other girls laughed – a little too enthusiastically, perhaps.

'Will you stay though, please?' asked Tracy.

I nodded, and sat down in my former seat. The magazine I had been reading was still open where I had left it. I picked it up again. Mum continued to beguile the girls with tales of kidnapping and torture, only now they didn't seem to have the same effect on the little salon's staff as before; they were coming to the end of their first lesson in how to handle dementia patients.

I thought about how much I had been enjoying my beer when all this excitement had occurred, and I suddenly remembered that I had left half a pint on the table across the road. I stood up and looked over at the pub. My companion was still sitting there, and next to him was my glass. I watched as he stood up, folded his newspaper carefully, and placed it under his arm. Then he looked furtively up and down the road before, very casually, picking up my pint, raising it to his lips, and draining the lot. Wiping his lips with the back of his hand and issuing a satisfied belch, he wandered off.

Mum was still chattering away in the background to the girls in the salon, about murder and mayhem at home, but I wasn't listening, I was more interested in the bloke across the road and my precious, stolen pint.

Eventually Tracy completed her work. Considering the difficulties, she had done a lovely job. Mum looked great.

'I'm going to give you a tip, Barbara,' she said to Tracy, as she put on her coat.

'Oh, thank you, Rose,' said Tracy, smiling.

I don't suppose Tracy made much money as a hairdresser, and tips were always welcome.

Mum opened her purse, thought about something for a moment, then leaned closer to Tracy. The hair stylist, sensing mum was going to say something confidential to her, leaned closer to mum as well. Their faces were almost touching.

'I want you to be careful with blackheads,' said mum.

Tracy stopped smiling.

'I see you have a big one on the side of your nose there,' whispered mum. 'Don't squeeze it or it will leave a mark.'

Mum nodded confidentially to Tracy, and shut her purse with a snap. She was often very helpful like that with total strangers.

10. The Recurring Drama

LIKE A GREAT MANY Alzheimer's patients, mum had fixed and recurring ideas. Once one of these random thoughts insinuated itself into her head, you couldn't shift it with dynamite; now ingrained into her consciousness, it would keep popping up at inconvenient moments. Eventually, it would fade away – until the next time.

I used to imagine these ideas as being like a person swimming underwater. The surface of the water represented mum's consciousness. Every so often, the swimmer had to come up for air. As soon as the swimmer broke the surface, the idea appeared in mum's mind and she would express it to the people around her, or perform some function or action associated with it. When the swimmer dived back below the surface, the idea was hidden away again. The time between 'breaths' could be weeks, days, hours, or minutes.

One of mum's most persistent notions was that of the little girl in the radiator. Mum didn't seem to think the little girl was in there all the time; she could go for days without referring to the radiator at all. Then, suddenly and without warning, the little girl would be there, and mum would engage with her until the episode played out, before going back to ignoring the radiator for a while.

I didn't know where she got the whole idea from, but I could cope with it so it didn't bother me too much. There was another such notion which was far more inconvenient for me, and it was that she would feel, from time to time, that someone was breaking in to the house. This only manifested itself when the sun was going down, and only then for a few days in a row before it disappeared until the next time. Unfortunately, while it was there it led her to shut every window and door in the house – even the internal doors – and lock those that she could. Worst of all, she would press down the little button – the 'snip' – on the internal Yale lock on the front door, so that the door could not be opened, even with the right key. This locked me out of the house. During one particular week, I returned from work to find myself locked out every evening.

The first time this occurred, it was pouring with rain.

'Mum!' I shouted through the letterbox. 'It's raining, open the door!'

'There's no-one here,' came the reply.

Only an Alzheimer's patient would shout that.

'*You're* there!' I shouted back through the letterbox. 'I just heard you speak!'

It all went very quiet.

'Mum open the door, it's tipping down!'

I could see her moving about in the hallway through the frosted glass in the front door, but she was making no attempt to let me in.

'Mum!' I shouted through the letterbox again, as the rainwater ran down my neck. 'Open the door! Please!'

'I can't!' shouted back mum. 'It isn't safe!'

'Yes it is! It's *me*!' I shouted. 'Of course it's safe!'

It was no good. The idea that she shouldn't open the door had become fixed in her mind, and no amount of persuasion from me was going to get her to see things any differently.

'Is everything all right?' I heard Mary's voice call from behind me.

I stood up and turned around. She was sitting in her wheelchair in the hallway of her bungalow – she'd obviously heard the shouting.

'Mum's locked me out, Mary,' I said, 'and she's put the snip on the door.'

'Oh dear,' sighed Mary. 'Shall I phone her?'

'If you would, that would be great, thanks.'

Mary picked up the telephone in her hall, and rang mum's number. Our telephone started to ring, I could hear it outside. I was getting soaked.

I saw mum's shadowy figure move across the frosted glass in the front door, and pick up the receiver.

'Hello,' said mum.

'Rose, it's Mary, next door.'

'Oh, hello Mary,' said mum. 'How are you?'

'I'm fine thanks, Rose. Can you come to the front door, please?'

'Okay, Mary,' agreed mum.

She put down the telephone and walked to her front door, then just stood there.

I waited in the rain motionless, and Mary sat in her hallway with the telephone receiver halfway between its cradle and her ear. No-one moved; the seconds ticked painfully away. The water was running down my neck.

'Rose…' said Mary again, but mum wasn't near the telephone now.

'Mum,' I called through the letterbox again.

'Yes!' shouted mum.

I looked through the letterbox: mum's eyes were staring out at me from the other side.

'Mum, open the door!' I said.

'I can't, it isn't safe,' replied mum.

'Mum, go back to the telephone, Mary wants to tell you something that's important.'

'Okay,' said mum.

Mum went back to the telephone and picked up the receiver again.

'Hello.'

'Rose, it's Mary,' said my patient neighbour, still sitting in her hallway. She was now getting wet too, as the wind drove the rain in through her doorway.

'Oh, hello Mary, how are you?' asked mum again.

'Rose, I'm fine. Rose would you like to come over for a cup of tea?'

'That would be lovely,' said mum. 'When shall I come over?'

'Come right now,' replied Mary.

'Okay,' said mum, and she put the telephone down.

I heard the snip on the Yale lock click upwards, and the handle turn. The front door slowly opened. I stepped quickly into the hall.

'I'm bloody soaked!' I said.

'You should have an umbrella with you on a day like this,' replied mum. 'I'm just going over to Mary's for a cup of tea. I won't be long.'

She wandered down the drive, and into Mary's house.

I smiled at Mary, and she smiled back.

'Come on in, Rose,' I heard her say. 'I'll put the kettle on.'

I went into our house to dry off.

* * * * *

The following evening the same thing happened.

'Mum let me in!' I shouted through the letterbox.

It wasn't raining this time, but my sheer frustration at having to repeat this scene again made it seem even worse. The *déjà vu* of living with an Alzheimer's patient drives you mad. You absolutely *know* something silly is going to occur, because a particular situation has happened before, and history starts to slowly repeat itself. You are caught in the middle of the drama, you know the way the scene ends, but you are quite powerless to change the outcome.

'There's no-one here!' shouted mum. I felt like trying to smash the front door down with my head.

'*You're* in there!' I shouted, again through the letterbox, remembering my line.

I say 'line', because it is like being an actor in a play. The Alzheimer's patient leads and directs the drama, and everyone else plays their parts, reading from an unchanging script. You end up thinking you're living in some fifth dimension; it's like the *Twilight Zone*, and it's *always* a repeat.

'Is everything all right?' asked Mary, right on cue.

I looked at her and forced a neighbourly smile.

'She's locked me out again, Mary.'

'Shall I phone her again? That worked last night.'

Mary, playing her part.

'Thanks very much, Mary,' I said. 'I'm sorry about all this.'

'Don't mention it,' she said. 'At least it's not raining tonight!'

I could hear the telephone ringing inside our bungalow.

'Hello,' said mum, picking up the receiver.

'Hello Rose, it's Mary.'

'Oh, hello Mary, how are you…'

I felt like I could scream.

'I'm fine thanks, Rose. Would you like to come over for a cup of tea?'

'Oh, that would be lovely Mary, when shall I come over?'

'Come on over right now, Rose. I'll put the kettle on.'

'Okay.'

The front door opened.

'Hello son,' said mum, as she passed me in the doorway. 'I'm just going around to Mary's for a minute, I won't be long.'

I waved conspiratorially to Mary, and she waved back. I entered the house.

Final curtain falls, and play ends. Take a sodding bow, Slevin.

I took the next morning off work and waited patiently for a locksmith to arrive so I could have the Yale taken off the front door, and replaced with a lock that didn't have that little snip. That had spiked mum's guns: she couldn't lock me out any more. He was at the house for about 25 minutes and charged me £90, but it was worth every penny.

I arrived home that evening with a spring in my step. I knew the drama of the previous two evenings could not repeat themselves. I was feeling very clever and pleased with myself, in a smug sort of way. Without my guile, the whole business could have gone on and on until either time ended or my head exploded, whichever came first.

I put my key into the new lock, and… crash! The door wouldn't open. Mum had put the chain across and outwitted me. I felt like running down the road screaming.

'I can't get in mum,' I shouted through the opening. 'Let me in!'

'It isn't safe!' shouted back mum.

They say the line between sanity and madness is a thin piece of string. It is, and I was walking its length like a man on a circus tightrope.

'Shall I put the kettle on?'

Mary was skipping her lines, but I was grateful for it.

'Thanks, Mary,' I called back.

It's hard to explain to someone who has never experienced it exactly what it's like to go through this process. It's a bit like watching a movie you've seen before, only this is much more intense because you're actually *in* it, right at the centre of the action, and, try as you might, there's not much you can do to change the way the story unfolds. Sooner or later, this starts to mess with your head, and you begin to wonder where it's all going to end. It's almost as though you lose the right to self-determination, you no longer have freedom of choice over your actions, everything is pre-destined; your role has been written, and all you can do is go along with it until the credits roll. As I think I may have said before, Alzheimer's makes everyone crazy.

I was muttering to myself like some sort of demented madman as I forced my little screwdriver to extract the two screws holding in the safety chain on mum's front door. There was a wild determination about my movements. Just getting into the house after work had become a battle of wills, and it was a war I was determined to win at all costs. When the safety chain had been removed, I breathed a sigh of relief. Now there was no way she could keep me out.

But although the drama repeats, there's no law against ad libbing.

* * * * *

The next night I came home with a sense of renewed vigour. I put my key in the door, no resistance, no chain, and I smiled. I pushed the front door open, and… crunch!

The door opened about three inches and stopped abruptly. I couldn't believe it.

'Mum, the door's stuck!' I shouted through the letterbox.

No answer.

I flicked up the letterbox lid and looked inside. I could plainly see the back of one of our kitchen chairs, which had been propped at an angle against the front door.

You can change the script, but so can the patient; as you improvise to derail the train, so they improvise to save it. Measure and counter-measure, tit-for-tat. Mum had made the house safe again, at least in her own mind, and I was back to square one.

'Mum, can you hear me?' I shouted. 'The door's stuck!'

'There's no-one here!'

The solution to our little recurring drama came quite unexpectedly.

Mary called out from behind me. 'Martin, the kettle's on, shall I call her now?'

'Yes, please Mary,' I sighed.

'What's she doing now?' asked Mary.

I looked through the letterbox.

'She's waiting in the hall for you to ring her. She's waiting for the telephone to ring!'

Then something happened between Mary and me. We both realised at once that the last sentence was very important, and was somehow the key to the whole mystery.

It began to dawn on me that the roles were clearly defined in our little play with three parts. Mum was the main character, I was the villain and Mary was the hero, riding in to save the day. And just as Mary and I knew our lines, so did mum. In her mind the key elements of the scene were:

1. Mum somehow manages to bar the front door before
Martin arrives home.
2. Martin arrives home and cannot get in.
3. Shouting occurs, which mum ignores.
4. Mary telephones mum.
5. Mum opens the door and goes to Mary.
6. Martin enters the house.

So she followed the sequence every single time, and not until she received her cue from Mary (the telephone call) could she open the door. She was merely being faithful to the script we had developed between us.

'I've just had a brilliant idea!' said Mary, beaming a huge smile at me.

'Yes?'

'What if I was to phone your mum half-an-hour *before* you're due home from work?'

I realised at once the beautiful simplicity and perfection of Mary's solution.

'That way, she would already be in here when you got home, so the door wouldn't be locked, and you wouldn't be locked out!' said Miss Marple, triumphantly.

Problem solved!

We tried this, and it worked like magic. If I'd been a bit smarter and realised this myself earlier, I could have saved £90 on the locksmith.

We simply cut a few lines of dialogue and rewrote the running order:

1. Mum somehow manages to bar the front door before Martin arrives home.
2. Mary telephones mum.
3. Mum opens the door and goes to Mary.
4. Martin enters the house.

My advice to anyone who finds themselves in a repeating drama with an Alzheimer's patient like this is to try and think of the whole episode as a play. Try and recognise the roles of the characters involved, including your own, and then think of a way to bring the curtain down before the normal time – removing one or two of the plot twists, as it were. Try to bring the final stages nearer to the beginning, so you effectively cut out the trauma in between. Of course, this is all a lot easier said than done, but the solution is inside the problem; all you have to do is become detached enough to see it.

11. The Man In The Grey Macintosh

I HAD BEEN CONSCIOUS for some time that I had been treating my mother like a prisoner. I would go off to work in the morning, lock her into the house for her own safety, and she'd be there until I came home in the evening. Later on I would go to bed, and again I'd lock her into the house. Apart from occasionally telling random hairdressers that she was being held captive, mum never complained. But she had been a very active woman in the period before her Alzheimer's, and I knew she missed going out and about.

One thing she had always liked to do was to hop onto the train on a Saturday and go the two short stops up the line from Coventry to Birmingham. Birmingham's market had been famous in the 1960s and 1970s, and the hustle and bustle always seemed to inspire her to new heights of shopping frenzy. She would dash about the covered stalls, laughing and joking with the stallholders, haggling here and there, and generally having a great time. She could spot a bargain at 100 yards, as keenly as any hovering falcon ever tracked a mouse. Then she and dad would come home on the train again after the market had closed, both laden with their bargains, happy as a couple of school kids.

It was a Friday night and we were watching television in the lounge. 'Mum,' I said. 'Would you like to go to Birmingham market tomorrow?'

I knew full well what the answer would be.

'Oh, I would *love* that!' she cried, in genuine delight. 'We could take Bonzo with us and go on the train!'

I thought about the difficulties I might encounter on the train journey, as I tried to keep an eye on mum, without having the added trauma of trying to prevent our demented dog from humping the leg off some terrified passenger.

'I think we'll leave Bruno here, mum,' I said. 'He doesn't like to go on trains.'

I had no idea whether or not this was true, but I didn't much care.

Bruno sat up straight as soon as he heard his name mentioned. 'Oh, look at him!' said mum. 'He wants to go shopping with us!'

'No, he doesn't.'

'Oh, bless him!' cried mum.

Bruno was looking at mum, then back at me, then again at mum. Of course, mum took these quizzical canine glances to mean that he really wanted to go on a train and have a look round the market where he could buy himself a bone and a new collar. And that he was promising faithfully to behave himself.

'He'll be *so* disappointed if he doesn't go,' pleaded mum.

'No, he won't.'

'Oh, he will. I understand him more than you do,' she said.

'No, you don't. He doesn't understand what we're saying, and he isn't going.'

Mum threw her arms around Bruno's neck as though he were a long lost relative.

'Poor Benji!' cried mum. 'I'll bring you back a new collar and a big new bone!'

Mum bent her head and kissed the hairy hound long and hard on the top of his head.

'Oh, bless him!' she cried again.

'We'll need to make an early start in the morning,' I said. 'We'll have a quiet day shopping.'

The next morning I got up at eight o'clock and mum met me, washed, dressed and ready in the kitchen. She had her hat and coat on, and was holding Bruno by his lead; a small piece of paper was attached to his collar.

'What's this?' I asked, taking a closer look at the paper.

'It's his name and address, just in case he gets lost in the crowds, then someone can take him home for us,' announced mum triumphantly, obviously very pleased with her idea.

It was some street in Dublin.

'I told you last night, he's not coming with us,' I said. 'And that address is in Ireland, anyway. Now, I'm going to get some breakfast.'

'Yes, of course it is,' she said. 'It's *our* address.'

I sighed as I poured the cereal into the bowl. 'No, it isn't, we don't live in Dublin. We live in Coventry.'

Mum looked at me as though I was becoming very forgetful, more to be pitied than argued with. She laid her hand gently on my arm.

'Yes we do, Richard. I think you need a holiday.'

I sloshed the milk into the bowl.

'My name's not Richard, and we don't live in Dublin. I *could* do with a holiday, though.'

Mum and Bruno went and sat together in the front room. Mum was very quiet; I think she was wondering who I might be, if I wasn't Richard.

Eventually, I got dressed, took Bruno's lead off and managed to get mum out of the front door without him. We parked the car at Coventry train station and headed into the main concourse.

'Two return tickets to Birmingham New Street, please,' I said to the man behind the glass wall at the ticket counter.

'Is the sea calm today?' asked mum.

'I have no idea,' replied the man. He looked somewhat surprised; given that Coventry is right in the centre of England, and is about as far as you can get from the sea in any direction, I didn't blame him.

'I'm not a very good sailor,' explained mum, to the ticket seller. 'I always get seasick on the ferry. I just wondered if it was going to be a rough crossing to England, that's all.'

'You're already in England,' replied the man, very quietly.

Mum nodded, and smiled, but clearly didn't understand. The man slid the tickets under the glass partition.

'Thanks,' I said, and we moved away. It gets very tedious explaining to everyone you meet that the person you are with has Alzheimer's. After a while you just stop bothering and leave them to figure it out for themselves, if they can – and, if they can't, who cares anyway?

'When's our train due in?' asked mum.

I looked at one of the display screens overhead.

'About 15 minutes,' I said.

'Let's have a nice cup of tea,' suggested mum.

In the small cafeteria we ordered two teas and mum ordered a jam doughnut, which she carefully wrapped in a paper tissue and placed in her handbag.

'Why are you saving the doughnut?' I asked.

'It's for Billy,' she said.

'Why don't you just feed him dog food? I'm sure he's not supposed to eat jam doughnuts and cream cakes, and all the other crap you give him. No wonder he's mental.'

'He is *not* mental!' cried mum. 'We love our mid-morning cream cakes. We both look forward to it.'

I bet he did; he'd really landed on his paws. I could just tell that this simple trip to the market was going to turn into a major adventure, like the simple trip to the hairdresser's.

The train was more or less on time, and we had finished our tea when it pulled into the station.

'Let's have a meal on the train,' said mum. I think she was trying to make the most of her day out.

'We can't,' I replied. 'We're only going two stops... we'll be there in less than 20 minutes.'

'It takes longer than that to get to Dún Laoghaire,' said mum, chuckling at my naivety. Dún Laoghaire is the port in Dublin where the ferry departs for Holyhead.

'Where do you think we're going?' I asked.

'We're going to England, aren't we?' said mum.

'We're *in* England, mum,' I said. 'We *live* in England. We've lived in England for *decades*. We're going to Birmingham market, that's all.'

'Oh,' she said, disappointed.

'And we're not going on the ferry, we're only going two stops on the train!'

Mum was nodding. 'Yes, that's right,' she said.

The Saturday morning trains to Birmingham are always crowded, and you're lucky if you can get a seat. I knew we probably wouldn't be able to sit together, so I decided to let mum sit while I stood nearby so I could keep an eye on her.

We boarded the train after a little queuing up.

'Stay close to me,' I said. 'I don't want you to get lost.'

'You don't have to worry about me,' said mum, indignantly. 'I know what I'm doing, you know.'

We squeezed down the narrow aisle of the first carriage, between the settling bodies and the two rows of seats. I was leading, and calling back over my shoulder. 'Stay close now,' I said, 'there's a vacant seat up here, you take it and I'll sit over here.'

We reached the seat. 'You can sit here, mum,' I said, turning around.

She wasn't there.

'Shit!'

I looked frantically back down the way I had just come, the way I thought we had both just come. I couldn't see the end of the carriage as people were still standing in the aisles and throwing luggage onto the overhead racks.

I started to roughly barge my way back down the train.

'Hey, steady on!' complained someone as I bumped past.

Suddenly the aisle was blocked in front of me by a big fat woman in a red hat. I didn't have time for courtesies, I had to get past her and find mum right now. This huge woman was actually standing in the middle of the aisle rooting through an enormous handbag.

'Wait a minute, I know I put it in my bag this morning,' I heard her say to someone as I drew level with her.

When I was small my dad had always insisted on me having good manners, especially when dealing with grown-ups, authority figures, or females of any age. 'Manners cost nothing, son,' he used to say. I hope he would have understood. I drew level with this mountainous woman, as she was still rummaging through her bag, when I simply took as big a step as I could, sideways.

'Oooooh!' shrieked the woman, as she crashed headfirst back into her seat, the contents of her handbag rattled across the metal floor of the train.

'Sorry!' I muttered as I went past her.

'Some people have no manners these days!' she shouted after me.

I couldn't see mum anywhere. A whistle blew and the train pulled away. I looked frantically out of the carriage windows, one after the other, hoping to God I didn't get a last glimpse of mum on the platform. I couldn't see her. As the train left the station, people melted away from the aisle into their seats, and I could see the whole of the carriage. I stood in the middle, desperately scanning the faces and heads about me. I couldn't spot her anywhere.

I began to make my way down the carriage, retracing our steps. I scanned every head and face as I passed. No luck. I came to the end of the second carriage, and still couldn't spot her.

Where the hell can she have got to? I thought to myself.

It suddenly occurred to me that she might have entered one of the small toilets which can be found at the end of each carriage. I went back down the aisle and found a locked cubicle.

'Mum?' I said, gently tapping on the door.

'I ain't your mother!' came back a deep male voice.

'Sorry!'

I turned again and went down the aisle towards the point where we had boarded the train, again scanning all the heads and faces as I passed. I entered the second carriage again and began to walk slowly down the aisle. If she wasn't in the toilet, and she wasn't in the second carriage, then she must be in this one, I reasoned.

She wasn't there.

I suddenly had a sick feeling: she mustn't have got on the train at all. We must have become split up on the platform back at Coventry. I boarded the train, and she didn't. If that was the case then she would be wandering around the city right now, completely lost, and I was already miles away and going in the opposite direction.

But I'd been *sure* she had boarded the train right behind me. On the fast train, it's only two stops from Coventry to New Street, the other being in the middle at the National Exhibition Centre. The NEC is a huge arena where thousands of people flock from all over the country to events like the British Motor Show and big rock concerts. Years ago I'd been there to see The Who and David Bowie.

'Next station stop, National Exhibition Centre,' announced the voice over the Tannoy system, and the train started to slow down. People began to get up from their seats and gather their bags together. Suddenly, I was plunged back into the middle of a mass of people, and I still had no idea where mum was.

I pushed and shoved my way roughly down the aisle again through the barricades of bodies. I was starting to panic. People were pulling down large and small cases, and squeezing down the aisle as best they could. Dozens of people were getting off the train here, and there was a large queue of others massing on the platform waiting to take their places on the train.

When the departing crowd had got off, and the new lot had boarded, I had dozens of fresh heads to scrutinize up and down the carriages. Everyone had changed and I had to start all over again looking for mum.

The whistle blew, and the train lurched suddenly forward, and then began to pick up speed. The next stop would be Birmingham itself, if I didn't find her by then I would be in a terrible mess: the train was heading up to Manchester after that. Frantically, I scanned the people on the NEC platform as we pulled away from the station.

Then I saw the back of her head.

I recognised her immediately by her clothes. The weird thing was, she was walking arm-in-arm along the platform with some bloke in a grey raincoat and black trilby. I couldn't believe my eyes – they were chatting as though they had known each other for years. Then they disappeared together around a corner, and I lost sight of them. It was too late. I was now on my way to Birmingham.

I stood there gazing out of the window like a man in a trance. I knew I had seen her, I just couldn't quite believe it; just in case I'd been mistaken, I did as quick and thorough a search of the whole of the train as I could, racing through each of the carriages before we got to Brum in the next 10 minutes. Some people looked up at me as I passed, others ignored me. What a variety of people we have in this country! People of all skin shades and hues, hair types, textures and lengths, cuts and colours; and what a mixture of body types, from the scarily skinny to the frighteningly fat, with all degrees of body mass in between. Every single bodily feature of every single person is slightly different; it's amazing how nature can manage to create so many variations on a single theme. As I passed through the carriages, scanning the river of heads, like a great sheet of bubble-wrap, all I could see were noses: big noses, small noses, long noses, short noses, fat noses, squashed noses, upturned noses, broken noses, bent noses, button noses, noses with warts, noses with freckles, and, in one case, an adolescent nose with an index finger stuck up it to the second knuckle. I had never really looked at people like this before.

I covered the whole length of the train, knocking on all the toilet cubicles on the way, and by the time the voice over the Tannoy announced 'Birmingham New Street, next station stop!' I had assured myself that mum was nowhere on this train. It had to have been her I'd seen.

As soon as we pulled into the station, I was first off. I ran to the information desk. 'When's the next train back to the NEC, please?'

The man looked at a screen over his head. 'Platform two, just leaving.'

I dashed up the stairs and ran along the corridor that runs over the platforms until I came to the staircase that leads down to platform two. The train was just pulling out when I managed to open a door – thank God, this little local train didn't have automatic locking – jump in, and crash the door shut behind me.

A quiet day's shopping, indeed!

* * * * *

As the train rattled back to the NEC all I could think about was the man in the grey macintosh.

Who the *hell* was he? I had only caught the briefest glimpse of him, and only from behind, but I was reasonably sure I'd never laid eyes on him before. He reminded me of a character in an old black-and-white film from the 1950s; in his long raincoat and black trilby he was dressed like Hollywood's idea of what a British spy was supposed to look like. But he could be anybody. He could be some sick weirdo who goes around the country kidnapping elderly women, but what for? For money? Most old people don't carry that much cash on them, and I made sure mum never did. For *sex*? Oh my God, the thought of it!

For what, then? Maybe he was just some perverted psycho who travelled the country, up and down the train network, collecting old ladies? I suddenly had the most bizarre picture pop into my head, of a huge barn somewhere in the middle of nowhere full of scores of elderly women, all wandering around in circles talking to each other whilst this shadowy figure in a grey mac and black hat watched it all from a high balcony, rubbing his hands with glee and laughing maniacally.

'And now, my dears!' he shouts ominously, from the high parapet, his arms outstretched to his captives milling below. 'Now, we are going to play *bingo*!'

I had to snap out of this. Like I've now doubtless said several times before, Alzheimer's sends the whole family crazy and it does an especially good job on the main carer.

'Next station stop, the National Exhibition Centre,' came the metallic announcement. 'National Exhibition Centre, next station stop. Passengers wishing to depart the train at this station, please make sure you have all…'

I stopped listening. As the train squealed and hissed to a stop, almost everyone seemed to stand up. The aisles were immediately blocked again. I waited as patiently as I could for the queue to meander towards the doors, and eventually stepped out onto the platform. I went the way I thought mum and the mysterious man had gone about 25 minutes earlier. The crowd milled towards the exits, and we began to move like a great herd of cattle towards the central complex of the NEC itself.

I noticed that most people were making their way towards the exhibition halls, and we passed a great sign which swung on wires over our heads:

FRANCHISE AND SMALL BUSINESS EXHIBITION

Everyone seemed to be going there, so it made sense for me to follow. If mum wasn't in there, and had left the NEC complex with that man, I was stuffed; there would be no obvious way of tracing her.

The crowd began to thin into a long line as we approached the entrance of the exhibition hall. When I reached the front I was asked for my ticket.

'Sorry, I don't have one, I'm just looking for my mother, she's lost.'

'Eight pounds please.'

The man collecting the tickets didn't care about my lost mother, I wasn't going in without either a valid ticket, or paying the admission charge. I paid him.

The NEC exhibition halls are massive and hold thousands of people; it was going to be a nightmare trying to spot mum amongst them. The one thing I had going for me was the man in the black hat, if she was still with him. Men rarely wear hats in Britain now, so he should stand out from the crowd. Over the main arena was a long balcony, and there were a number of bars and restaurants on the first floor with large windows overlooking the exhibition floor. I decided to make my way up there – then I could look down on the crowd for a black trilby hat. This seemed like a good plan.

I shoved through the crowd going up and down the staircase, then I shoved through the crowd on the upper landing, then I shoved through the crowd to the bar area, where people were chucking down tasteless, overpriced beer in plastic glasses, oblivious to my anguish. No sign of mum in here. I shoved my way through the crowd again, back out of the bar and along the main balcony. When I got to the main barrier, I was able to look down on the crowd milling below.

The Franchise and Small Business Exhibition was spread across three huge halls, and I was looking down onto a sea of heads that swirled around the stands in only one hall. I scanned the jostling horde from one corner of the great complex to the other, wondering if I'd ever pick out the man in the black trilby hat.

No, was the answer.

The river of heads ebbed and flowed around the stalls and swirled down the aisles, forming patterns and shapes as the crowd intermingled, separated, and mingled again. It was fascinating watching the crowd from above like that; all individuality was disappearing as the herd instinct took over, and all these people, who couldn't possibly know each other, moved like a single organism. *Blood cells moving through an artery*, I thought.

I went back down the stairs to rejoin the throng. I felt in my bones that mum wasn't in that hall, but that didn't mean she wasn't in one of the others. I swirled with the rest of them along the aisles and through the large portals separating one giant hangar from the next. I had not realised that so many people might want to start up a small business. Here there were franchises to be bought for pretty much any type of business you could imagine. For £20,000, I could become a loss adjuster for the insurance industry; or an accident specialist, photographing catastrophes at the roadside; or I could travel the country repairing scratched paintwork on cars, taking stone chips out of windscreens, or pulling the dents out of car panels. I could train privately to become an accountant or a vet; or I could open a shoe shop, a dress shop, a wedding gown hire shop; or I could sell power tools. I could learn to repair televisions or computers, or I could learn to steam clean carpets and curtains for anyone who would like to employ me to do so.

I wondered what mum had already signed up to; I could imagine her sitting at a desk with a slimy salesman saying, 'You're never going to regret this, Mrs Slevin, your new career as a freelance travelling tree surgeon will be very rewarding indeed.'

I had better find her quick.

In the second hall the crowd was even bigger than that in the first. I pushed and dodged through the crowds, looking at the people sitting at the stands, the people milling about, the people standing around, the people moving up and down the stairways. I looked at everyone, and really saw no-one.

Then, out of the corner of my eye, I saw him!

It was the man in the grey coat and the black trilby hat. He had just exited this hall and was heading into the third exhibition. I only got a glimpse of his back, but I was *sure* it was him. I started to shove through the throng, closing on him with every step. I pushed through the gateway into the third hall, and looked about. He had disappeared. Where was he? He was here just a second or two ago. I forced my way forwards frantically, and then I glimpsed him again. He was carrying two cups of tea on a plastic tray over to one of the stands. I followed him, and he laid the tray down on a table. He gave a cup to a woman in a red baseball cap, put a cup down for himself, and sat at the table. When I approached, I recognised the woman in the red baseball cap as mum.

'Oh, Richard!' said mum, as I approached. 'There you are. I'm going to start a business embroidering baseball caps for people! Isn't that great?'

Mum's bright red baseball cap had the word 'Rose' embroidered across the front in fancy gold lettering.

I took a very deep breath.

'How do you do?' said the man in the grey macintosh. 'You must be Richard.'

I shook his hand. 'Actually, my name's Martin,' I said. 'My mum thinks that I'm her brother sometimes, he's Richard. She has Alzheimer's.'

'Ah,' he said, 'I thought it was Alzheimer's. My late wife had it, so did both my parents.'

He stirred his tea thoughtfully.

'It runs in families, you know,' he said. 'I suppose I'll get it too, one day. I wondered when someone would show up to claim your mother.'

'We got separated on the train,' I explained.

'Easily done,' he remarked. 'I realised she was lost, so took her along with me. I realised someone would turn up for her sooner or later.'

'Thank you, that was very kind of you.'

'Not at all,' he replied, putting his cup down. 'And don't worry about the new business embroidering baseball caps. I made sure she didn't sign anything, or give them any money. Even if she did, I don't think they'd be able to hold her to it.'

'No, they wouldn't,' I replied. 'We've had that trouble before with some double-glazing people.'

The man in the grey macintosh nodded. 'Are you looking to start up a small business, or secure a franchise, perhaps?'

'No,' I said. 'I was just chasing my mother. We were supposed to be going to New Street market, but mum got off the train a stop too early.'

'Ah,' he said.

'What about you?'

'I retired a while ago from the military. I served 22 years in the Army. I've got a good pension, don't really need the work, just thought I might find something interesting to occupy myself with. Getting bored at home, that's all.'

I nodded.

There was a silence for a few moments, and then he smiled at me. 'Your mother's been telling me that you're a bullfighter for Coventry Council,' he said. 'That sounds interesting.'

'She tells people that,' I said. 'I don't know where she got that one from.'

Actually, I suspected it was from the television. The phrase 'Mad Cow Disease' had been in the papers a lot lately, and there were news reports about it on the TV fairly regularly. I guess that mum had simply taken a few extra mental steps to give me this somewhat exotic new job.

He nodded. 'It's a fascinating disease, Alzheimer's,' he said. 'My wife thought I was dead. She used to talk to me and all that, but then she'd tell people that I had been blown up in the war. She used to cry about it sometimes, even when I was sitting on the sofa next to her.'

I shook my head. 'By the way,' I said, 'I don't think it is hereditary, you know. Just because your parents had it, doesn't necessarily mean you will, too.'

(This is true; the Alzheimer's Society says that in more than 99% of cases heredity is irrelevant. The major risk factor is simply age.)

'Oh, I think it is,' he replied, as though it were a certainty. 'Trouble is, I'll never know if I have it or not, will I?'

I shook my head. 'No, everything will seem the same to you.'

We fell into a silence again.

'I was thinking!' announced mum suddenly. 'I could put the machine in the conservatory, then I could work out there.'

'What machine?' I asked.

'The machine for embroidering my baseball caps, of course,' said mum. 'Look!'

She pulled the red baseball cap off her head and thrust the front of it at me.

'Very nice, mum.'

'It says "Rose" on the front!' she said, excitedly. 'The man did that for me.'

'Yes, I can see that.'

'Well, I must be going,' said her latter-day knight.

'Let me pay you for mum's ticket,' I said, taking out my wallet.

'Not at all, I wouldn't dream of it,' he replied, gallantly. 'Besides, she's very good company.'

'Well, let me buy you a drink, or a sandwich or something,' I asked.

'Actually, I was thinking of having a drink before I went,' he said, relenting.

'Great,' I said. 'We'll all have one.'

The three of us adjourned to a small bar not far from where we were sitting.

'I'll have a whisky, if you don't mind,' said the man.

'I'll have a whisky too!' piped up mum.

'You've never drunk whisky in your life!' I said.

'Oh, yes I have!' she said, indignantly. 'I always have a whisky at bedtime.'

This was completely untrue. Her annual intake of units of alcohol had always been close to zero, and even at family weddings or parties she would only ever have one small glass of sherry, for as long as I could remember.

'Right,' I said.

I started to move towards the crowded bar counter.

'Make them large ones!' she called after me.

At the bar I ordered two large whiskies – taking care to put some water into mum's. I had a beer.

Mum and the man in the grey macintosh chinked their glasses together to seal their new venture. Mum seemed to have got the idea into her head that this man and she were going into business together.

'Cheers,' said the man, and knocked his back in one.

'Cheers,' shouted mum, and did the same.

The man reached over and lifted up mum's baseball cap. 'The street kids wear them like this,' he said, turning it around so the peak was sticking out of the side.

Mum smiled.

'Well, I really must be going,' said the man. He shook hands with both of us, doffed his hat to mum, in a very gallant and gentlemanly way, and disappeared through the crowd. It occurred to me then that I didn't even know his name. I still don't, sadly.

'Let's have another!' said mum, and thrust her empty glass at me.

Alzheimer's patients can often exhibit dramatic changes in character like this.

'Don't move from here!' I said, collecting her glass and heading for the barman.

'I won't,' she said, leaning on the bar-rail like she was a regular at this.

I came back with another whisky and water; mum snatched it off me and downed it like Wild Bill Hickok.

'Time we were going!' I said, and we moved towards the exit. I held her by the sleeve all the way back to the train station.

The train was not nearly as crowded on the way back. We found two seats easily, and within a minute of sitting down mum was fast asleep, her red baseball cap crushed against the side of her head and the back of her seat.

And as we rattled and swayed our way back to Coventry, I thought about the man in the grey macintosh, his wife and his parents, and all the other sufferers of Alzheimer's disease that we never hear about, but who struggle on, day after day, coping with a condition that no-one in power seems to be doing very much about.

12. Making The Decision

I HAD BEEN CHATTING to Heather one night on the net, and had rashly invited her around to the house for a bite to eat, and to meet mum. The day she was due to come over it occurred to me that maybe I should do something about the décor in our house.

I stood on a kitchen chair and started to remove the rows of socks from the ceiling; carefully withdrawing the small pins so as not to chip the paint or plaster. We had got into a routine, mum and I, with this sock thing. I would take a pair down, wear them and then put them into the washing basket. Mum would wash and dry them, and then pin them back to the ceiling or a wall.

'Can we start to put my socks back into my sock drawer like we used to, mum?' I ventured as I stood there, painstakingly removing them. 'It's better, don't you think?'

'I don't know,' she said, predictably. 'Ask Peggy. She's the one who puts them up there.'

'Aunt Peggy says she'll put them back in the drawer from now on,' I said.

I was learning how to play this game.

'That's all right then,' replied mum.

When the socks were all put away I went into the lounge to dismantle the Christmas tree: after all, it was the middle of February.

'What are you doing?' cried mum.

'I'm putting the tree away until next Christmas,' I said.

Mum put her hands to her face and started to weep. 'Please don't,' she sobbed.

I put my arm around her, trying to comfort her. 'We can't leave it up all the time, mum,' I said.

'Why not?' she said.

A good question, when you stop to think about it.

'People just don't,' was the best I could do. 'A Christmas tree is supposed to be just for Christmas. People take them down again afterwards.'

'It's so pretty,' she said, ignoring my argument. 'Turn the lights on.'

I switched on the dozens of little coloured lights. Mum stared at the sparkling tree. She never really paid any attention to the tree when the lights were off; but when they were lit she would just stand and stare at it for long periods, lost in the land she now inhabited. It was a bit like the way people tend to stare into the flames of a real fire.

'It's magical,' she observed.

Alzheimer's seems to have a way of compensating its sufferer for the carnage it inflicts on their everyday memories. It often leaves them with childishly fresh eyes, which bestow an infantile wonder upon creation, as though they were observing life for the very first time. Little things the rest of us take for granted they see with a new and enchanted vision, discovering charm and wonder everywhere in this tired and unfair world of ours. Perhaps the new vision is not so much a corrupted sense, but a heightened or sharpened one; perhaps there really *is* magic left in the little things still, but the rest of us do not have the terrible affliction of Alzheimer's and therefore have become immune to the spell. Sadly, the compensation for the damage is a passing phase, whereas the wreckage is permanent, and on the whole the exchange of new eyes for old memories is a terribly unfair one.

'Okay, I'll leave the tree up,' I said.

Bruno was now a part of our family, and he had his little ways too. He would run out into the back garden and wait for me to come out to him. This was a game he enjoyed. I would run at him (a few brief steps, as the back garden was not large) and clap my hands, whereupon he would bark and run into another corner of the garden and wait for me as before. Then I would clap my hands and chase him again. He would keep this up for a good half-an-hour. Of course, poor Bruno didn't know that this game was designed to give him some exercise; I had stopped his nightly walk down the street for a while, being too embarrassed to be seen out with an Alsatianish mongrel with a shaved bottom. But his rump was no longer piglet pink, and was now a sort of misty grey, like a five o'clock shadow: designer stubble for dogs. I'd have to start walking him again, I thought.

It was around this time that a worrying incident occurred. I was awoken one morning around 5am by a very loud and persistent knocking on the front door. I jumped out of bed, hurriedly put on my dressing gown and went to the door. I remember being surprised to discover it was not locked.

I opened the door to see a man standing there whom I instantly recognised as Joe, a guy I'd gone to school with 35 years earlier. Mum was standing beside him, dressed in just her nightie. She was holding a strappy sandal in one hand. I braced myself, as the air was freezing.

'Hello, Martin,' said Joe. 'I found your mum wandering around the shops down there.'

He jerked his head to indicate the row of small shops at the end of our street.

'She seems quite confused,' said Joe. 'I thought this was the house.'

'Come inside, mum,' I said. 'Thank you very much, Joe. I appreciate this.'

'Ah, it's nothing,' said Joe. 'I was going to work anyway.'

A quick wave and he was gone.

'Sit by the fire, mum,' I said. 'You'll freeze to death out there dressed like that. What did you think you were doing?'

'I was looking for the shoe man,' she replied, starting to shiver. 'I need to get these sandals fixed.'

She held one of them up. The ankle strap had been sliced through cleanly. I didn't have to guess who had done it, and it wasn't me or Aunty Peggy.

This incident brought the harsh reality of our situation home to me. The truth was simple: I just couldn't cope.

I wasn't in the house often enough, or long enough, to supervise my mother properly. Even when I *was* there, like now, she still wasn't safe. Mother could not live at home any longer. I'd known this decision was coming, but that didn't make it any easier. I tried to tell myself that it would be for the best, that she would be much better off if I could find her a place somewhere where they could take care of her properly; that she would be safer there, happier. As I said earlier, we can get used to almost anything. I also think we can find ways of justifying anything, too, if we try hard enough. My mother had always been the first to help whenever anyone she knew had ever needed support; now, she was the one who needed help, and all she had on her side was one stupid, useless son. The guilt I felt at this time was overwhelming; she had never given up on me, but here I was giving up on her. It was all so bloody unfair.

That afternoon, with a heavy sense of defeat, betrayal and weakness, I telephoned the social worker who had contacted me months ago to ask me if I needed support when mum had first been diagnosed.

'No, I'll be fine,' I had said back then, without even thinking about it.

How wrong I had been.

'I'll come out next week and have a chat,' she said cheerily.

* * * * *

Mum was still staring at the Christmas tree when Heather knocked on the door.

'I've brought you both some supper,' she announced as she came in. 'Home-made lasagne. I hope you both like it.'

Mum and I just thought it was Christmas all over again. She ate as though she hadn't had a proper meal in weeks, which she probably hadn't. My cooking is basic at best, whereas Heather's was sensational. Mum set about the dish with a frenzied zeal, eating a huge portion and then going back for more – something she never did with any of my offerings. She usually talked through a meal, too, but tonight she was silent. She simply ate and ate, until the whole dish was empty.

'That was wonderful, Wendy,' she enthused.

'My name's Heather,' said Heather, though she appeared not to be in the least offended.

'I never knew you could cook like that, Wendy,' remarked mum.

'I'm a chef,' she said – which explained the quality of her cooking. 'And my name's Heather, Rose. I'm not Wendy.'

Mum nodded as though she understood.

'You've put on an awful lot of weight since I saw you last,' she said, sagely. 'You really should get more exercise.'

'Thanks,' replied Heather, smiling.

Strangely enough, this was the start of a great friendship between my mum and Heather. Mum continued to call her Wendy every time they met, and even Heather began to think it was funny in the end.

A few days later the social worker called at the house to speak to us, and an era for my family drew to a close.

The social worker was a pretty, middle-aged woman with a genuine smile, an unconquerable sense of humour and an observant manner.

'How are you keeping these days, Rose?' she asked.

'I'm doing great,' replied mum, emphatically.

'That's good. The last time I talked with your son, Martin, he said you were a little confused sometimes. Is that still the case?'

Mum looked perplexed. 'But you couldn't have talked to Martin,' she said. 'He lives in Africa.'

The social worker looked at me. I shrugged: there's your answer.

'This is Martin,' said the social worker, pointing at me.

'That's not Martin,' laughed mum. 'That's my brother, Richard.'

The social worker shook her head. She didn't have to play along with mum's delusions like I did. 'No, Rose. That's your son, Martin. He's been looking after you.'

Mum shook her head. 'I don't need anyone to look after me. I can do everything myself.'

'But you know this is, Martin, though. Don't you?'

'I don't know who everybody is in here,' said mum. 'This house is more like a hotel than a home. There's always people coming and going. I don't know who half of them are.'

'I see,' said the social worker, turning towards me. 'Do you want me to start looking for a place for your mum to stay?'

So this was it. If I said yes, there would be no going back.

I looked at mum, and she just sat there, oblivious to the fact that her entire future was about to be decided. I nodded. I couldn't bring myself to say the words out loud.

The social worker closed her folder and smiled. 'I'll see what I can do,' she said, standing up from the kitchen table. 'I'll give you a call next week.'

We shook hands formally, and she left.

'She was nice,' I said to mum, when the lady had gone.

'Who was she?' asked mum.

I felt my face get suddenly hot. 'She was someone from the council,' I said. 'She came out to make sure that you're okay.'

Mum nodded and seemed satisfied with the explanation. But something about the social worker had unsettled her. She was very thoughtful thereafter for a couple of days, and each evening when I came in from work I found myself locked out of the house again, a kitchen chair propped under the handle.

That recurring drama was still being played out, but only in runs of a day or two and often with several months between episodes. This time she had a new motive.

When I complained that she was locking the door, she replied, 'I have to. I have to protect myself!'

'From who?' I would shout back, in exasperation.

'From those who want to put me away,' she would shout back.

'No-one wants to put you away,' I would argue, feeling the guilt sweep over me like a tidal wave.

'Ah, you don't know everything,' she would reply. 'I hear things. People tell me things. They warn me. They tell me to protect myself.'

'Who tells you these things?' I once asked her, trying to reason with a mind that now worked to its own rules, and not to the world's.

Mum would look at the radiator quickly, and then look down at the floor.

'The little girl in the radiator?' I said. 'She ought to mind her own business.'

I couldn't believe I had actually said that.

'She knows things,' whispered mum.

I changed the subject, and got on with the business of life in our house, until the next evening, when the entire performance would be repeated, often blow for blow, and word for word.

* * * * *

About a week later, I got a call from the social worker, who gave me an address of a care home which specialised in cases of dementia. She asked me to drive out at the weekend and give the place the once-over.

I asked Heather if she would come with me. She and I had started seeing each other properly now, and although we'd only been together for about a month by then I had quickly come to trust her good judgment and solid sense.

We agreed to drive out together the following Sunday afternoon and found a large, isolated house, standing on a small hill overlooking the road. As we turned into the driveway, the abandoned mansion in the film *Psycho* came to mind.

'Looks charming,' I said.

'Let's take a look inside,' said Heather.

We walked up the long flight of stone steps to the front door, and rang the bell. I was expecting someone like Lurch from *The Addams Family* to amble down the dusty hallway, but the door was swung aside by a young girl in a smart, blue and white uniform.

'Good afternoon,' she said, brightly. 'Are you visiting a resident?'

'We're here to view the place,' I said. 'My mother might be coming to stay here.'

I realised I was lowering my voice as I spoke; I think I subconsciously felt embarrassed to admit that I was committing my mother to a home.

'I'll get the manager for you,' replied the nurse. 'Do come in.'

We were shown into a long hallway, and asked to wait. The house was spaciously designed with sculptured plasterwork on the ceiling, and had obviously belonged to someone of some wealth or importance a couple of hundred years ago. I imagined it was the kind of place that once had live-in servants; today it was a functional care home for unfortunates like my mother.

A silver-haired woman of about 60 walked up to us. 'Hello,' she said, shaking hands with us both. 'I'm Sally. I understand you'd like to look around?'

110

'Yes, please,' I answered, feeling as guilty as hell.

Sally began the guided tour, walking us down a long corridor and waving her hand into various rooms, as though she was pressed for time: 'This is the dining room. This is the television room. This is the kitchen.'

We popped our heads briefly through each doorway as we passed. The empty dining room was laid out like a small café, with a few tables here and there draped with plastic covers. A small, blue and green plastic cup with a lid and spout and two handles had been left on one table. It was like a baby's training cup: I wondered if it was for a resident.

Heather looked into the television room. An elderly lady was sitting alone watching football on the TV. 'Hello,' said Heather. 'Sorry to disturb you.'

'Fuck off!' shouted the old lady.

I popped my head in.

'You fuck off too!' she shouted.

'Pay no attention,' said Sally. 'That's Alice. Everything all right, Alice?'

'Fuck *off!*' shouted Alice.

'We'll leave her to it,' said Sally, and the three of us all toddled off to view the kitchen.

Large stainless steel units were placed around the walls. There was little to see, but it looked clean enough.

'Breakfast is at eight, lunch at 12, and dinner at five. Bed by 10,' said Sally. 'We have a dietician who puts the menus together, and a trained chef who prepares the meals.'

We nodded.

'Let's look at some bedrooms,' suggested Sally. 'We can go upstairs.'

We followed Sally up a very narrow and very steep flight of stairs. 'My mother would have trouble with these,' I said. 'They're very steep.'

'It's an old house,' replied Sally, 'but there is a small elevator for residents who are unsteady on their feet.'

Once upstairs we wandered down another long corridor. On the wall outside each bedroom door there was pinned a small photograph of the relevant resident, together with a hand-written note of each name.

'This one is vacant at the moment,' said Sally, throwing wide a door. On the wall outside was a photograph of an old man wearing a woollen hat and no teeth. The note said simply: 'Charlie'. I wondered what had happened to him.

Charlie's old room was pretty basic. The top half of the walls was painted a pale green, and the bottom half a grubby cream, and there was a single bed, a bedside table with a lamp on it and a small dressing table.

'The bedrooms are all singles,' said Sally, 'but they're quite serviceable. There is a private bathroom, as well.'

Sally opened the *en suite* bathroom door. A wet room yawned before us: no bath, just a slanting, tiled floor, where Charlie would stand to wash himself, the suds and dirty water running away through a hole in the floor. There was also a toilet and washbasin.

'Are all the rooms the same?' asked Heather.

'Yes, they're all the same,' said Sally.

An old man had shuffled into the room behind her. He was wearing a frayed dressing gown and had a box of dominoes in his hand. Sally turned around.

'No, Fred!' said Sally, in a very commanding tone of voice. 'Charlie isn't here any more, is he?'

Fred looked a little perplexed.

'Charlie can't play dominoes with you today, Fred,' announced Sally, still in a loud voice. 'Now run along and find someone else to play with.'

Fred shuffled from foot to foot, not sure what to do next.

Sally took the old man by the shoulders and physically turned him through 180 degrees so that he was facing the door again. 'Off you go, Fred,' she said.

'Dominoes today, with Charlie,' muttered Fred, as he shuffled away down the corridor.

Sally watched him go and then returned her attention to us.

'Any questions?'

We both shook our heads, too shocked to speak, and then we drove home in complete silence.

13. A Memorable Sunday

WITHIN A FEW WEEKS Heather had moved in. Neither of us were spring chickens any more – we were both in our late 40s – and not under any illusions, but when it's right, it's right, and we decided not to waste time. There aren't many women around who are willing to try to make a go of it with a middle-aged man they've just met, and his 80-year-old mother with Alzheimer's. I always admired Heather for that.

One Sunday morning we were going about the business of becoming fully awake, mooching around the kitchen trying to decide what to have for breakfast and which paper to read first. Mum was in her dressing gown, with odd socks and odd slippers on, talking to the little girl in the radiator, Heather was pulling out drawers here and there to see where everything was kept and I was feeding Bruno in the conservatory.

'Let's have a traditional Sunday roast for dinner today!' said Heather, suddenly. 'We can have roast beef, Yorkshire pudding, stuffing, the works… how does that sound to everyone?'

I must admit, after my awful cooking, it sounded fantastic.

Mum clapped her hands together in glee. 'Oh, that would be wonderful, Wendy! We haven't had a proper Sunday dinner for ages.'

I hung my head in shame and pretended not to hear.

'Bruno really likes roast beef and Yorkshire pudding,' announced mum confidently, as though the mental mutt actually ate it every weekend.

'That's settled then,' declared Heather. 'Dinner will be at one o'clock sharp.'

Mum skipped into the living room and put the television on. Bruno, having heard his name mentioned, skipped across the kitchen looking for a treat, and I skipped out of the way.

Heather really is a great cook, and, in what seemed like no time at all, our little kitchen had been transformed into a hive of industry.

Potatoes were peeled and sitting in a pot of water, a great slab of beef was seasoned and prepared, and various clumps of vegetables were being spread out on the kitchen work surface. The oven was on, and things were happening. When you live on egg and chips, or fast food from the local takeaway, a real home-cooked meal can become the highlight of your whole week, as many a student living away from home will testify. I had done my best for mum, culinarily-speaking, but my best was not very good.

In fact, as I look back now it's hard for me not to criticise most of what I did for mum. My shortcomings stare back at me reproachfully through the mists of time, and they make me uncomfortable. I suppose I'm not alone in this. At the time, the very business of everyday living gets in the way of thinking too deeply about things; we muddle through and do the best we can. But as we look back at our lives, most of us think we could have done better – we could have been kinder, less severe, more perceptive, more in tune with the needs of others, more forgiving, more patient, a little more chilled out. In my defence, the sad truth is that no-one is ever shown how to be a carer. There's no training. When you step in as a carer, Social Services are grateful – you're taking a great financial and logistical burden away from them, and they tend to let you get on with it. This may be the greatest fault with the system – amateurs like me are left to manage these situations without help, support, training or even encouragement. I realise now that this lets both the patient and the carer down badly; but nothing will ever change until people and politicians are made more aware of the constant needs of an Alzheimer's patient. So I don't entirely blame myself. I know I could have done better, but that's life; I have a feeling of nostalgic melancholy I have learned to live with.

Anyway, as Heather bustled about the kitchen that Sunday morning, everything in my garden was coming up roses. Mum's spirits were buoyant, Heather was happy, I was happy, and Bruno was behaving himself. What could possibly go wrong?

'What can I do to help?' asked mum.

'You could lay the table for me, Rose,' replied Heather.

'I can do that,' announced mum, and she started to take the cutlery out of the drawer.

'Everyone seems to have a job but me,' I said to Heather.

'Everything's perfectly under control,' replied Heather. 'You don't need to do anything.' Then, as an afterthought: 'You can take Bruno out for a walk if you want? He's getting in my way.'

Bruno had realised that something sensational was happening in the kitchen, and he had been sniffing around Heather, trying to be her best friend ever since she had unwrapped the lovely joint of beef and seasoned it on the kitchen work surface.

His shaven hair had all-but grown back: a walk was in order.

'Come on mate, let's take a trip around the block,' I said, rattling his lead. Bruno was at the front door immediately, whining to be let out.

'We won't be long,' I called back to Heather, as the dog and I slipped out of the front door.

It was too early to go to the pub, so we headed for the park. The great, green expanse spread out before us like an ocean, we had the whole place to ourselves. I let Bruno off the lead, and he ran and ran. Some dogs seem to just run for the sheer joy and exhilaration of it, and Bruno sped along the grass, handlebar ears pinned back by the wind. It was a joy to watch him, as he tore around me in a giant circle, then ran off and came back, and raced away again. Dogs do seem to get tremendous pleasure from the simple things in life; I remember standing in the middle of the park that Sunday morning, watching Bruno and wishing – in that respect at least – that I could be more like him at times.

Eventually, he came back, with his tongue hanging out of the side of his mouth, panting like mad, and lay on the grass beside me. He had run himself to a standstill. I put my arm around him and gave him a cuddle. Although Bruno could drive us all crazy on occasions with his little eccentricities, his presence in the household had done my mother a world of good, there was no denying that, and I was very grateful to him for it.

After a while, I clipped his lead back onto his collar, and we began a slow walk back to the house. Sooner or later, I knew, Bruno's owner was going to sort her life out, and when that happened she was going to want him back. I knew I would miss him when he went, and I wondered what sort of effect the return to his rightful owner would have on mum's condition. Maybe we could get a dog of our own? Perhaps a puppy that mum could raise during the day when she was in the house on her own? Perhaps if we did that she wouldn't need to move out to a home? Now Heather was living with us too, she would have to be involved in the decision making process as well. I wondered as we walked back to the house, if Bruno missed his owner, and if so, would he miss us when he went back to her?

'We're back!' I called, as we ambled through the front door.

'I've laid out the table,' announced mum, proudly.

Bruno and I went in the kitchen to look. There were only the three of us going to eat that afternoon, but mum had laid out four places – probably because our little kitchen table had four chairs around it. Arranged neatly around each of the serving places were three spoons, making twelve spoons in all, and no knives or forks.

'That's nice, mum,' I said.

Mum beamed.

'Mum's finished laying the table,' I said to Heather.

'Have you seen it?' she replied.

'Yep. I'll change it when she's not looking,' I said.

The dinner was almost ready, and Heather was busying herself with the final preparations. Bruno sat in the kitchen, leaning against the washing machine. It seemed as though his run in the park had tired him out; he had his eyes closed, and he looked half asleep.

'Bruno's very sleepy,' observed mum as she came in and out of the kitchen. 'What's the matter with him?'

'Nothing. He's just tired from his run in the park,' I said. 'Leave him while he's quiet.'

She went back into the lounge to watch TV, and Heather checked on the dinner. I smiled as I looked at Bruno. He really did look to be asleep; sitting upright, leaning against the washing machine, swaying very slightly to and fro with his eyes closed and breathing deeply, he looked quite comical. We even started to whisper, so as not to wake him. Bruno opened one eye and looked at me, and then closed it again: it was a long, slow, winking movement, unhurried, almost in slow motion.

Strange dog, I thought to myself. 'Is there anything I can do to help?' I asked Heather.

'Just fix the table,' she replied.

I took some knives and forks from the cutlery drawer and cleared all the extra spoons away from the dining table. Then I went into the lounge to sit with mum for a while until the dinner was ready. It was an idyllic Sunday afternoon, and the smells of roast beef wafted through the rooms of our small bungalow like a tantalising perfume.

Mum and I passed the time away in the lounge watching nothing particular on TV until dinner was ready. Bruno continued to doze in the kitchen, leaning against the washing machine.

Mum had been speaking to the little girl in the radiator more and more lately, but when I questioned her about it her responses were cheerful and upbeat. Her time spent with the little girl was more pleasant these days, and they chatted together about all sorts of things, mainly about events from mum's childhood, and she usually seemed to come out of these engagements feeling happy, although at times this was tinged with melancholy.

What about that puppy idea? Could that work? I didn't want to send her away to a strange place where she wouldn't know anybody; could she stay at home if a puppy gave her something to look after and focus on? But I had to face two facts. The first is that Alzheimer's is a degenerative disease which only goes one way – from bad to worse. I was kidding myself if I thought I had the time and expertise to give mum the quality of life at home she really deserved. The second was that she was in no position to take on the responsibility of caring for a puppy. She couldn't even look after herself. A puppy's welfare would have to be taken into consideration as well.

It's easy to avoid a painful decision in life if you can find an excuse to postpone it. We all do it, and I was no exception. I was scrabbling around for ways to keep mum with me, and the puppy idea was just another way of avoiding the inevitable; but in my heart

I knew that she had come to the end of the road at the bungalow. She didn't even recognise the house as hers any more, so leaving it would not be a great hardship for her; she probably wouldn't even miss it.

'Dinner's almost ready!' called Heather from the kitchen.

Mum and I followed that most wonderful of British aromas, fresh roast beef, into the little kitchen. I noticed immediately that Bruno had not roused from his half-unconscious state by the washing machine, but continued to sway gently with the measured tempo of his own breathing, his eyes still closed.

I shook my head when I saw him like that again. Most dogs would surely have roused at the thought of some stray titbit falling to the floor by now; maybe there was really something wrong with him?

Heather was dealing out portions of roasted vegetables onto the three plates she had laid out along the work surface. Roast potatoes, Brussels sprouts, cabbage, sage and onion stuffing, and perfect Yorkshire puddings were all evenly spread out, awaiting the hot, sliced beef.

'Can you open the back door, please?' asked Heather. 'It's as hot as hell in here.'

The little kitchen always became uncomfortably warm when the oven had been on for a while.

Bruno opened one eye carefully, and shut it quickly again – I am certain of it.

'Sure,' I replied, and opened the kitchen door which led to the conservatory. So that the conservatory windows didn't become wet with condensation, I went through and opened the back door which led onto the small rear garden. There was now a clear run from the kitchen to the garden.

They say that, to those involved, car crashes can appear to take place in slow motion. Time itself seems to slow down as the impact becomes inevitable, probably because the brain functions speed up as nature's way of giving us a final chance to react and survive. I remember re-entering the kitchen that Sunday and the same thing happening to me.

As I put a foot inside, Bruno launched himself from his supposed doze into the air, with the instant reactions of a gun-shot sprinter. His two front paws hit the kitchen work surface and his head leaned forward – all in perfect synchronicity. His jaws opened wide, and my heart sank.

'Aaarrrggghhhhh!' screamed Heather, as the dog's famously satanic growl boomed around the little kitchen. He barged past me, through the kitchen door, through the conservatory and out into the garden, free and clear.

Heather, mum and I stood open-mouthed, looking at the empty metal roasting pan, where only seconds ago our lovely joint had been resting.

'He's got the beef!' wailed Heather.

I instinctively ran after the dog, with Heather and mum hot on my heels. Heather still had the large carving knife and fork in her hands.

Bruno sat at the top of the garden, facing us. His handlebar ears seemed to be stationed at an even more acute angle to his head, making him look somehow guilty, angry and sorry, all at the same time. He still had the whole, steaming hot joint of beef in his mouth, and he was continuing to let out that unearthly growl of his, telling us to keep well away.

The three of us formed a line at the bottom of the garden. The Sheriff's posse had cornered the outlaw, and the stand-off began; Bad Boy Bruno wasn't for giving up. It was a delicate situation.

'Isn't he very naughty for doing that?' said mum. 'You're. A. Very. Naughty. Boy!' She wagged her finger at the dog very deliberately in time with every word. I remembered the same voice and manner from my childhood.

'*Do* something!' demanded Heather, nudging me with her elbow.

Bruno lowered his head and dropped the joint onto the grass. Great streams of saliva dribbled from his mouth onto the meat. He laid a paw on the joint and rolled it around for a bit, before taking a bite from it. Bits of grass and clay were already sticking to its surface.

'What do you want me to do?' I said. 'Even if I manage to get it back, we can't eat that now.'

'You're. A. Very. Very. *Very*. Naughty. Boy!' mum wagged her finger at the dog again. 'And. I'm. Not. Going. To. Talk. To. You. Any. More!'

Bruno lowered his head and mum walked back into the house.

Heather looked at me and sighed, and then followed her back into the kitchen. I could hear Heather crashing and banging about inside, pots and pans were being thrown into the sink with a determined violence. I was left in the garden staring at this strange dog who I'd come to love. He wagged his tail at me, and picked up the joint again. It was covered in bits of grass. I couldn't help but smile. I think he was trying to show me how clever he had been. Bruno had lulled us all into a false sense of security with his little game; I was sure he had planned to steal the meat all along, and was only waiting for some poor sap to open the back door for him. I never realised a dog could be that smart.

The atmosphere in the house had changed slightly. Frosty might be a good word to describe it. No-one spoke. Heather simply put more carrots and cabbage onto each plate, and the three of us silently sat down to our now vegetarian Sunday lunch.

To describe it as a bit of an anti-climax would be a huge understatement. Bruno was locked out in the garden for the rest of the day by mum, and we watched television, a solemn, silent trio, until bedtime. Bruno was eventually allowed back inside at around 10 o'clock.

'You. Go. To. Bed. And. Just. Think. About. Your. Behaviour!' said mum, wagging her finger at the dog again. Bruno slept in the hall.

Unfortunately, that wasn't the end of the story. When I woke up to the sound of my alarm clock the next morning, Bruno was in bed with me.

'What the hell...?' I said as I poked the hairy hound in the back, trying to work out what had happened in the night. Bruno rolled over to face me and yawned, his breath smelled of roast beef.

Where was Heather?

I got up and dressed and found her fast asleep on the sofa in the lounge.

'What's going on?' I said.

Heather pulled the blanket down off her face and sat up.

'I got up in the middle of the night to use the loo,' she said, 'and when I was in the bathroom, Bruno got into the bed with you. When I came back, he wouldn't let me get back into bed. He kept growling at me. I had to come out and sleep here. You were snoring for England!'

My new girlfriend wasn't happy.

'Something has to be done about that dog!' she announced. 'Take him to obedience classes.'

'I did, but he shagged the instructor,' I said, helplessly.

Heather threw me a disgusted look, flopped back down on the sofa and pulled the blanket over her head. That was the end of that conversation.

14. The House With The Green Kitchen Floor

ABOUT A WEEK LATER, and out of the blue, I got a call from my Aunt Ellen in Dublin.

'Martin,' she said. 'I've been thinking about your mammy an awful lot lately. I've been dreaming about her, too. I feel as though I ought to come over and see her…'

She let her words trail away.

'You know you're most welcome to come over and stay any time at all, Aunty Ellen,' I said.

'Good,' she replied, 'because I'll be there in the morning.'

'Oh, right…'

Ellen always was the decisive one. She gave me the details of her flight from Dublin, and I agreed to meet her at Birmingham airport the following day.

'Mum,' I said, when I put the phone down. 'Aunty Ellen's coming to see you tomorrow.'

'I don't have an Aunty Ellen,' she said.

'No, but I do. She's your sister.'

'Oh, Ellen!' exclaimed mum. 'That would be wonderful!'

My mum and her last surviving sister had always been very close. Mum was six years Ellen's senior, and a special lifetime bond had developed between the two girls when they were small. Mum was in great spirits when she realised that the pal of her childhood was coming over.

I took her with me to the airport the next morning. After I pulled into the car park, I switched off the engine and turned around to face her, sitting in the back seat.

'Now listen, mum,' I said, trying to make my voice sound stern and authoritative, so that she would pay attention. 'I don't want any of your shenanigans in there.'

'What's that supposed to mean?' she replied, looking shocked.

'This is a big airport,' I said. 'There are thousands of people coming and going from all over the world, all the time. I don't want to have to spend the rest of the day trying to find you. I don't want you getting lost, so stay really close to me, okay?'

'When did I ever get lost?' said mum, in a hurt voice. 'I'm not a child you know.'

'You got lost when we went to Birmingham on the train,' I said.

'That wasn't my fault, I just got off at the wrong stop, that could have happened to anybody!'

'You got lost when you were wandering around the shops in your nightie.'

'That was a misunderstanding.'

'You got lost when you couldn't remember where we lived and ended up at Wendy's house.'

'I was *visiting*!' shouted mum. 'I'm not stupid!'

'I didn't say you were stupid, mum,' I said, trying to calm her down. 'But you do get confused sometimes, don't you?'

There was a pause.

'Sometimes,' she agreed, reluctantly.

'I just want you to stay close to me in the airport, that's all.'

'I will,' she said, and started to root through her handbag. This was her sign that the conversation was over, and she didn't want to discuss the subject any more.

I opened the car door and was about to step out when I felt her hand on my shoulder.

'Sit back down, Richard,' she said softly. 'Just for a moment. I want to ask you something.'

I shut the door.

'Am I sick?'

I hadn't expected that. The words echoed around the car. I didn't really know what to say.

'What makes you say that? Are you *feeling* sick?' I fumbled with the words.

'Sometimes I think I am,' she whispered.

'Why do you say that?'

She shrugged her shoulders and looked out of the window, but didn't answer. People in jogging bottoms and flip flops were dragging over-packed suitcases across the tarmac; a policeman was waving traffic around an intersection; people were milling around everywhere. They all looked as though they had their lives sorted out, they knew where they were going, or thought they did. I wondered how many of them would end up with Alzheimer's. All these focused people, moving today with determined strides, who wouldn't even know the names of their own children come that terrible day.

'You do get a little confused sometimes, mum,' I said.

'Do you think it's just my age?' she asked.

'Of course it is,' I replied.

Although mum spent most of her time thinking she was in her childhood again, at that moment she seemed to realise she was elderly; for a brief few moments, she seemed focused and in the present.

'Don't worry about it,' I said.

Mum nodded. 'That's all right then.'

I opened the car door again.

'Where are we going?' asked mum as we stepped out of the car. 'Anywhere nice?'

'We're not going anywhere,' I said. 'We're meeting your sister, Ellen, who's coming to see you from Dublin.'

'Oh, that's right!' exclaimed mum. 'I can't wait to see her!'

I linked her arm and we walked across the road and entered the main airport concourse under a large 'Arrivals' sign.

It was a Saturday morning, and the hall was already crowded with people waiting to meet friends and relatives on incoming flights. Professional drivers were standing around with placards, people trundled heavy cases on wheels and children chased each other around, screaming. The faint characteristic scent of aviation fuel filled the air.

'I need to check on Aunty Ellen's flight,' I said to mum over the hubbub, and walked us both towards an overhead flight display screen.

'I can't see her,' said mum, looking excitedly around.

'She's only just landed,' I replied. 'She won't be through yet. We need to wait over here.'

I led mum across the floor and we waited by the large double doors through which my Aunty Ellen would eventually appear.

'I still can't see her,' said mum.

'She isn't here yet,' I said. 'She still has to collect her bags. Keep watching those doors.'

'How long is she staying?' asked mum.

'She didn't say, she just said she was arriving this morning.'

Mum continued to look all around. Every young girl with brown hair that passed us, mum gave special attention to. I wondered if mum was expecting her little sister to be a child, too.

The double doors opened and people from Ellen's flight started to wander through.

'She should be in this lot somewhere,' I said.

Mum's interest was piqued instantly, and she started scanning the first of the group eagerly.

'Oh, Ellen!' she suddenly cried, and ran forwards with her arms outstretched. She flung her arms around a grey-haired lady in her mid-60s and kissed her on the cheeks, they hugged in the concourse. They rocked together in the embrace. An elderly man came up and stood quietly beside them, and I went over too.

'Mum, that's not Aunty Ellen!' I said.

The old man was smiling.

'What?' said mum, pulling suddenly away.

The elderly lady extracted herself with some difficulty from mum's fervent embrace, and grabbed the old man by the arm.

'I'm sorry about this,' I said to the couple. 'We thought you were someone else.'

The old lady nodded and smiled, but I could see she was still a bit startled. I led mum away by the elbow.

'That wasn't Aunty Ellen, mum,' I said. 'Wait until I see her.'

'She looked just like her!' said mum.

I sighed. 'It's an easy mistake to make.'

Moments later, my aunt actually did come through the doors. I recognised her immediately.

'There she is!' I said, pointing.

Mum ran over again and threw her arms around her sister, and then the two of them came over to me arm-in-arm so I could hug the aunt I hadn't seen in some years. Then mum hugged me, though I'd only seen her two minutes ago. Then everybody hugged everybody else again.

'I can't believe you're here!' exclaimed mum.

'Well I am here, so let's go and get a cup of tea,' said my aunt. 'I'm dying for a cup of tea.'

The three of us made our way out of the arrivals hall and back into the main concourse, where there were bars and shops scattered here and there.

'Let's go in here,' said Ellen, and we all trooped into a coffee bar.

'How was your flight?' I said, when we'd all sat down.

'Grand,' replied my aunt. 'I'm glad I made the decision to come over.'

My aunt looked at my mum as though she was trying to weigh something in her mind. 'How have you been Rose?' she asked.

'I'm fine,' said my mum. 'There's nothing the matter with me, it's just my age.'

'I'm glad to hear it,' replied Ellen, and she looked directly at me. My aunt leaned closer to me, and whispered, 'I want to have a chat with you, Martin, when we can have a minute or two to ourselves.'

I nodded.

Over the past year or so, Aunt Ellen had kept in touch with us by telephone. She would call at fairly irregular intervals, whenever the mood took her, and I had been appraising her of mum's worsening condition at each call. She was under no illusions.

I went up to the counter and ordered the tea. When I returned to my seat the two women were deep in conversation.

'...and if it wasn't for Richard, I don't know what I would have done lately,' said mum, turning and smiling at me.

'Richard?' said Ellen.

'Yes, Richard,' said mum, nodding in my direction.

'Oh, Rose,' replied Ellen, gently. 'This isn't Richard, this is Martin.'

Mum seemed confused.

'You do know that don't you?' pressed my aunt.

Mum nodded. She hated to think that she had made a mistake; if anyone challenged something she said, she would brush over it, as though it was of no importance.

'Of course I do,' said mum.

My aunt looked at me and smiled.

'So, how are things with you, Martin?' she asked. 'I hear you have a new girlfriend?'

'Yes, her name's Heather. She's living with us now.'

'That's a good thing,' replied my aunt. 'How is she getting on with your mammy?'

'They get on fine,' I said.

Suddenly mum got up from the table and went across to a young couple who were sitting at another table across the way from us. She appeared to speak to the girl for a moment, then to the boy, and then she sat down and joined them.

'What's she doing now?' asked my aunt.

'She does this a lot,' I replied. 'She sees someone and thinks she knows them. She just strikes up conversations with anybody. Most of the time the people don't seem to mind.'

Ellen was shaking her head.

'I have to watch her all the time,' I said, 'or she would just go off with anyone.'

'I can imagine,' said my aunt. 'How are you coping with her at home?'

'Not very well really,' I said, deciding to be honest. 'Heather helps, but really I think the time has come to find mum a place where she could be looked after properly.'

'I think so, too,' said my aunt. 'I'd take her myself, but we don't have the room.'

'It's not just about the room, Aunty Ellen,' I said. 'You can't take your eyes off her for five minutes. She leaves the iron on, the gas on, the doors open. Anything could happen. She thinks Heather is Wendy, she thinks I'm Uncle Richard, and she's living in a time in her childhood that I don't know anything about.'

'I'll have a talk with her,' replied my aunt.

The couple mum was talking to got up to leave, and mum got up with them. The three of them just started to wander away down the airport concourse.

'Where's she going?' asked my aunt.

'She's leaving with that couple,' I said. 'I'll go after her.'

I ran after them, and caught her by the elbow. 'This way mum.'

'Bye, now!' said mum to the couple, who smiled a little nervously at me, and hurried away.

'Time to get going,' I said, as we rejoined my aunt.

The journey home from the airport was uneventful, and when we reached the bungalow I introduced Ellen to Heather. They got on famously from the word go, and chatted for hours about everything and nothing, with mum joining in now and then with the odd story that sent everyone into fits of laughter. My aunt was very skilful at getting mum to talk about what was happening in her life, and she told me later that she thought mum was living in her mind in around 1940, when she had been 15 and Ellen nine.

'Do you remember that sweet shop on the corner of Bath Avenue, Rose?' asked my aunt. 'Our mammy used to take us all there every Sunday after Mass, and buy us a big bag of sweets each?'

'Oh, yes!' cried mum. 'We used to get them great big gobstoppers, and those sticky toffees… We used to look forward to it all morning.'

'Then we'd go home and we'd all have to mop that bloody horrible green lino floor in the kitchen,' laughed Ellen.

'But Richard didn't have to do it because he was a boy!'

They both chuckled at the injustice of that.

I hadn't really been listening to the conversation, but something in my mind clicked and I knew that what had just been said was important.

'The house had a green kitchen floor?' I asked.

'It was a great big kitchen, Martin,' explained Aunty Ellen, 'where we all lived when we were small. It had a green lino floor. You weren't posh if you didn't have lino in the kitchen in them days!'

The two women laughed.

'It was horrible really,' she said. 'No-one would want it now. You peeled it off a roll and just stuck it down, and all us girls had to mop the bloody thing every Sunday, or we didn't get the sweets.'

Mum and her sister were chortling at the memories which were carrying them both back over 60 years.

The house with the green kitchen floor!

I had assumed that mum was in some sort of fantasy-land, the details of which she just made up as she went along since the onset of her Alzheimer's, but she was only living inside her own memories… Memories probably long forgotten when she had been well. The phenomena of rolling back the rug, as the first consultant had called it all those years ago, had triggered images and thoughts long buried and brought them to the surface to be replayed again in full colour.

My aunt stayed just for the weekend, and flew home on the Sunday evening.

When we came to say goodbye to her at the departure gate, she turned to me; there were tears in her eyes.

'I'm so glad I came this time,' she sniffed. 'I don't think I'll see her again somehow, and if I did, she wouldn't know me.'

Mum, unconcerned, waved and simply said, 'I'll see you, Ellen,' as though they'd be meeting up again very soon.

Ellen gave me a hug. 'Look after Heather,' she said. 'She's a lovely person.'

Then mum's last surviving sister, her closest pal from the years they had spent as little girls in the house with the green kitchen floor, turned and, with a last wave, left her life forever.

15. First Home

PAINFUL AND DIFFICULT decisions tend not to go away just because we find excuses to avoid making them. You can put the event off many times, but one day you have to face it.

Our visit to that first nursing home had started the ball rolling, so to speak, but we were a good deal shocked by the place and we had put off the day when mum would have to move in there. We were supposed to have contacted the social worker after our visit to let her know if we wanted the spare bed, but we had failed to do so, and we assumed that now, several weeks later, there would be no spaces available. Mum was getting more and more forgetful at home, and simply couldn't be trusted to be by herself safely any more.

Heather worked as well, so it was just mum and Bruno in the little bungalow for most of the day. Locking her in there was both inhumane and dangerous.

We were reminded of the nursing home when the telephone rang one Friday evening. It was the social worker.

'I was just calling to see if you had made any arrangements regarding mum yet?' she asked cheerily; she made it sound as though it was *her* mum we were discussing.

'No, not yet.'

'Only, the reason I wanted to speak to you is because another vacancy has arisen there...'

Her words trailed away. I wondered who had died to make that space available.

'Okay, I'll speak to my partner and get back to you.'

'If you would, please... These beds are very scarce these days, you know.'

She rang off.

That night I spoke to Heather when mum had gone to bed.

Heather shrugged her shoulders. 'I was shocked by how bad some of those old people were. By bad I mean, how far gone...'

'I know what you mean,' I said.

'I felt so sorry for Fred,' she said.

'I liked Alice, myself,' I replied, and we both laughed.

'Your mum wouldn't like Alice,' observed Heather. 'I've never heard your mum swear.'

I thought about it. 'Neither have I,' I said.

'I wonder if all care homes are the same?' asked Heather.

'I don't know,' I replied. 'Maybe we should wait and speak to the social worker again? Maybe there are some other places we could go and look at.'

Heather was nodding enthusiastically. 'I'll speak to her again tomorrow.'

* * * * *

Throughout the whole of the next day, my mind kept returning to the visit of a few weeks before. I kept thinking about Alice – presumably someone's mother, and granny – plonked in a chair, alone in a room, with the telly tuned into some sports programme and the sound turned down.

Then there was old, threadbare Fred wandering aimlessly along corridors seeking out a dead friend: just one more forgotten old man, looking for someone to play dominoes with – not much to ask, really – while the staff turned him around and sent him on his way, instead of finding him someone else.

Then there was Sally, managing the place with a sterile, detached, disinterested, business-like attitude – as a farmer might manage a herd of cattle.

And then there was the place itself: the steep and, I thought, dangerous stairs, the clinical, surgical green walls, the photographs pinned to those walls – but for whose benefit? So the residents might recognise themselves and know which room was theirs? Or for the staff, so they might know who slept where? Or so that the occasional visitor might be able to locate their relative? I wondered.

During our brief visit, I remembered being struck by the fact that Heather and I were the only non-residents and non-staff members in the whole place. Where were all the other visitors? It was a Sunday, after all. When I became more used to the way these places work and are run, I knew that such establishments receive few regular visitors. The old – especially the old and demented – are quickly abandoned by their relatives. Once grandma's mind has become impaired to the extent that she exhibits extreme or very unusual behaviour, she is shut away to the regimented mercies of Sally and her colleagues. *Breakfast is at eight, lunch at 12, and dinner at five. Bed by 10.*

If an old person breaks a hip in a fall and goes into a regular hospital, on average they will receive three family visits per day. If the same old person is admitted to a care home, they will not receive three family visits per month.

I have never quite come to terms with these facts, but I think that, when the mind has gone, so to speak, there is a tendency to believe that the character of the patient, the inner nature and the personality, has gone, too. This is simply not true, and more efforts should be made to educate the public about dementia in general, and Alzheimer's in particular. The percentage of our population who have dementia in one form or another is terrifying, and yet little is said about it. No politician ever raises it as an issue, and no campaigns are fought on its behalf. Dementia in our society is a secret, social pandemic, which blossoms behind closed doors through ignorance and neglect, and it's about time someone stood up and said so.

* * * * *

'How did you get on with the social worker?'

It was the following evening, and I started to quiz Heather before I had even taken off my coat.

'There are no vacancies anywhere else at the moment,' she said. 'There is only the spare room we saw on that Sunday – apparently it's vacant again. She says if we really don't like it we can either keep mum at home or she could go into a hospital until a care home has a vacancy somewhere else. She said the place we saw isn't the worst one around. We need to give her an answer before next weekend.'

'Not the worst one around?'

'That's what she said.'

We began a heartfelt discussion which went on until the early hours of the next morning, as we swayed back and forth between putting mum into a hospital or the home we had visited and hated. Eventually, we agreed that we didn't want her to go into a hospital when she wasn't really sick – not physically, anyway.

'Maybe we could put her into the home for the time being,' I suggested, at last. 'Then if somewhere nicer comes up, later on, we could perhaps move her.'

Heather nodded, and we called it a night.

Thus are such momentous decisions made.

Heather called the social worker back later that day. It was suggested that we would take mum down to the home the following weekend. Once that was agreed there seemed to be no way back. It was almost as if I had agreed to commit a crime and now I couldn't back out of it, no matter what my conscience might be telling me.

The rest of that week was among the strangest of my life – not because anything bizarre or incredible happened, it didn't, but because I knew that at the weekend I was going to trick my mother into going into what was by any other name a mental institution, from where she would probably never emerge alive. That might sound melodramatic, but a care home for the dementia patient is the 21st century equivalent of the old Bedlam. The patients are treated with much more respect and dignity nowadays, true, and their rooms are cleaner, and they are fed properly; but madhouses they effectively are, no matter what we call them.

For mum's part, she continued to cuddle Bruno, talk to the little girl in the radiator, and listen to the Irish band with just as much devoted rapture as before.

* * * * *

I suppose it was my conscience bothering me, but I tried to make her final week at home as pleasant as I could. We sat in the front room every night and chatted away about everything and nothing.

She told me about her childhood in Dublin, about growing up in the house with Peggy, Ellen, Marie and Richard, her sisters and brother. She spoke about them as though they were all still alive, though Marie and Peggy had both been dead over five years. She spoke about the courtship she'd had with my father, and how happy they had been. Again, though, she spoke about him as though she had seen him only yesterday; and as she chatted, I thought about her rug being rolled further and further back. By now, I imagined, there was more carpet inside the roll than on the floor.

I think it was on the Wednesday that the conversation turned to the people she saw in the house.

'How is the little girl in the radiator getting on these days?' I asked.

'All right, I suppose,' came the distant reply. Whenever mum spoke of the little girl in the radiator, her voice became sadder and softer, and she drifted away slightly, as though she were trying to remember something that had become vague and distant.

'Is she still trapped in there?' I asked, gently.

Mum nodded slowly. 'She will always be trapped in there,' she said.

'Why is that, mum?' I asked. The strange and probably unique illusion that a child was trapped inside our domestic heating system had begun to fascinate me. I wasn't trying to become an amateur psychiatrist; I was just trying to get to the bottom of this one delusion, as it seemed the most peculiar, and persistent, of all.

'She has no way out,' replied mum, simply.

'Is she happy in there, mum?' I asked.

Mum lifted her face and looked at me. I saw a sadness in her eyes that I had not seen for a long time.

'How could she be?' she answered. 'How *could* she be?'

I didn't want to let this drop, and pressed on. 'How did she get trapped in there in the first place?' I whispered.

Mum shook her head. 'She doesn't know how it all happened,' she replied. 'One day she was happy at school, and then suddenly she was caught in there.' Mum nodded towards the radiator. Then she slowly ran her fingers along the rippled face of the heater. 'Ever since then, she's been trapped, and she can't get out.'

'What's it like in there?' I asked. By this time I was as engrossed in the story as mum herself.

'It's very dark,' said mum, softly. 'It's very dark, and she gets very frightened, poor little thing. And she's very lonely.'

'She still tells you things?'

'She speaks to me all the time,' said mum.

'What does she tell you?'

It sounds strange now, looking back, but mum and I had rarely communicated together at such a deep and personal level before, even though the subject of our discussion was a fantasy.

'She tells me secrets about Peggy, and the others,' she said, in a confessional tone. 'She tells me all sorts of things. Secret things.'

'What sort of secret things?' I whispered.

Mum shook her head.

'Can't you tell me?' I asked.

Mum shook her head again. My mother had always been good at keeping confidences. I remember when I was small her telling me once that a secret was a sacred thing, that it was like a precious gift that someone had asked you to keep safe for them, and that if a friend gave you such a gift it was because they trusted you. If you gave their precious gift away to someone else, if you betrayed that trust and told their secret, it was like stealing from them. I never forgot that, and became very discreet myself. Mum was keeping the secrets of the little girl in the radiator now. Alzheimer's doesn't change our personal values, they are too deep-seated for that; it only alters our perceptions, and messes with our memories. Who we are, at a fundamental level, remains unaltered.

'Okay, I understand,' I said.

Mum smiled.

'Does she ever tell you nice things?' I asked, trying to lighten the mood a little.

'Sometimes,' nodded mum, 'Not often, though.'

'What nice things does she tell you?' I asked.

'She tells me how good to me you are,' replied mum, matter-of-factly.

The words felt like a slap in the face. I must have blushed, something I haven't done in years, because I felt my face become hot. I couldn't stop thinking about the coming weekend.

'She tells me how kind you are to me,' said mum, smiling innocently.

'That's nice,' was all I could think of saying.

Heather and I decided to take mum out one evening for a nice meal before she went into the home at the weekend. We chose a restaurant we both knew which served great food, and I called them up and booked a table for three. I was a little wary about this trip out, as taking mum anywhere always involved a certain amount of risk, but I figured that, between us, Heather and I could deal with pretty much anything that might happen.

Heather selected one of mum's best dresses, one that was still intact, and helped with her makeup and brushed her hair; the finished result brought a lump to my throat. I hadn't seen her look so nice since dad had died. Alzheimer's patients tend to withdraw from the external world, so that things which once mattered 'out there', like personal appearance, suddenly no longer have meaning. Mum had let herself go since being diagnosed, and to see her all dressed up like this was really quite special for me.

'Where are we going?' asked mum.

'To a very nice restaurant,' replied Heather. 'We're going to have a lovely dinner.'

'Oh, that sounds wonderful,' said mum. 'Is he coming?' She nodded towards Bruno, who was sitting watching the proceedings in the hallway.

'No, they won't let Bruno in the restaurant, mum,' I said. 'He has to stay here and guard the house.'

Mum seemed to understand this. She nodded and said, 'Never mind, I'll bring you back a doggie bag, Bruno!'

We all laughed at the joke. The atmosphere was very light and jovial, and I wondered why we hadn't done this before.

We got into the car and set off. Bruno watched us go from the bedroom window.

The table was booked for 8.30pm, and it was only 7pm. Feeling the lightness of the occasion, I said, 'Let's have a drink first.'

We called into a local pub and the three of us stood at the bar. It was already starting to fill up with drinkers, and besides us there was a large crowd of men who looked like they had been drinking all day. They were singing rugby songs at the top of their voices, and enjoying themselves.

I bought the drinks, passed Heather hers and then turned to give mum the bitter lemon she had ordered. She was nowhere to be seen. Then I suddenly heard her singing. She was standing right in the middle of the rugby lads, singing some old Irish ballad, and they were all listening to her; no-one spoke, you could have heard a pin drop. When she had finished, they gave her a huge cheer and a round of thunderous applause. Mum finished off the turn by kissing every single one of them.

When the time came to leave they waved us a hearty farewell, and they all kissed mum again. She was having the time of her life.

We reached the restaurant dead on time, and the head waiter took our coats. Heather and I had eaten there before, and the waiter had often laughed and joked with us. When he saw mum he began by being very respectful, but as soon as he realised that mum was 'not quite right' his manner noticeably changed towards us. Maybe I was being oversensitive at the time, but I am certain that he thought mum shouldn't be there, and I found his attitude to be both insensitive and insulting.

We had a drink at the bar, and scanned the menu. The food sounded wonderful, and mum was unsure of what to have. The waiter came over, and asked us if we were ready to order.

'Not just yet,' I said. 'Can you give us a couple more minutes?'

'Certainly, sir,' he replied and went away. I noticed as he went, he cast a curious glance over my mother. I thought, *If he does that again,*

I'll say something to him. But then I reasoned that it was probably just my imagination, so I forgot it. Later, I discovered I wasn't being paranoid: Heather had noticed all of this, too.

He came over in a little while, and asked us if we were ready to order yet.

Mum asked him a question: 'Excuse me,' she said, 'is the salmon from Sainsbury's?'

Heather and I both giggled like a couple of school kids.

The man looked shocked. 'We don't buy our salmon from a supermarket, madam,' he replied, looking mightily offended at the very thought of it. 'Our salmon is caught in a Scottish river and shipped down to us the same day. All our produce is fresh and home-made.'

'Oh, I see,' replied mum thoughtfully. 'I'll have the pork chops, then.'

The head waiter blinked a few times in rapid succession, as though something had just landed in his eye. 'Very good, madam,' he said.

'Me name's Rose,' said mum.

He smiled at mum.

Heather and I ordered and the man went away. Over the next few minutes the three of us chatted in the bar as they prepared our table. I could see this waiter whispering to other staff members and sniggering; I was beginning to become angry.

Mum called the man over again. He stood next to her.

'Is it Christmas yet?' asked mum.

I think Heather began to sink a little lower into the plush armchair. The waiter began to blink as fast as his eyelids could open and close. He looked at me.

'My mother has Alzheimer's,' I said, although I shouldn't have had to mention it at all. 'She wants to know if it's Christmas yet. Perhaps you could tell her?'

By this time his eyes were opening and closing so quickly that I thought he was going to have some sort of seizure.

'No, madam,' he said, at last. 'It won't be Christmas for another nine months.'

'Oh, I see,' said mum. 'Thank you very much.'

As he went away, I thought how much nicer a person she was than he. Heather and I felt uncomfortable during the rest of the meal; we could hear them talking about mum, and looking over not too discreetly, though neither of us wanted to say anything. The head waiter didn't even come over to ask if we were enjoying our meal, something he had always done before.

I have wondered since why Alzheimer's makes some people so uncomfortable. Generally, the patients are great fun: there's no harm or malice in them, and they're almost never dangerous to others. Why, then, do they generate such fear? I think it's that it strips away the veneer of all personalities which surround it. That is to say, the best and worst character traits of each of us come to the surface when we are unexpectedly confronted by the condition in another. That may sound crazy, but I have seen it happen so many times. Nice people react with kindness and joviality; the not-so-nice react with cynicism and scorn. If they only knew the figures! If they only knew the percentage of the population over 60 that contracts Alzheimer's, they might not be quite so condescending; there is a world of confusion waiting patiently in the future for a great many of us, who today think we have life well and truly sorted out.

After the first course, mum had two desserts, a large bowl of jam roly-poly and custard, followed by a huge slice of Black Forest gâteau and fresh cream. At last we were preparing to leave and called for the bill. The head waiter came over to return my credit card.

'I trust sir found the meal to his liking?'

'We all enjoyed it,' I replied.

He smiled the kind of smile people give when they don't really mean it. It's as false and valueless as a two-tailed tuppence.

We got up to go. 'Shall we leave a tip?' I said to Heather.

'I think your mum already has,' replied Heather, looking down at mum's seat.

Mum had urinated all over the plush velvet covered chair. There was a huge, wet stain spreading across the pale beige, velvet seat. Heather and I just started to giggle, and by the time we got out of the restaurant door we were in hysterics of laughter.

'Well done, mum,' I said. 'That will teach them to be so silly.'

Mum looked at me; she was smiling a massive smile and looked really pleased with herself, as though she had just done something really clever.

The rest of that week is lost to me now. Nothing momentous could have happened, because the next thing I remember is Sunday morning. Mum came into her bedroom after breakfast and saw me packing a suitcase with her clothes.

'What are you doing?' asked mum.

'I'm packing your case,' I replied truthfully.

'Why?'

'We're going on holiday,' I lied.

'Oh, how lovely!' said mum. 'Is Wendy coming too?'

'Yes, Heather's coming with us. She'll be here in a minute.'

Mum clapped her hands, and did a little skip around like a delighted child. I have never felt more worthless in all my life.

'Will we be by the seaside?' she asked, her eyes wide in anticipation.

'Not very near,' I said.

Heather walked in.

'We're all going on holiday together, Wendy!' cried mum.

Heather and I looked at each other.

'Yes, Rose,' said Heather.

I carried mum's case out to the car, and mum sat in the back. As we drove away, Bruno was looking out of a bedroom window.

When we got to the home, I pulled in around the back, and helped mum out of the car.

'What a very grand hotel!' said mum. 'You shouldn't have got somewhere so posh. This must be costing a fortune!'

We rang the old-fashioned bell before the huge door. Presently, another young nurse admitted us and ushered us inside. The door was locked behind us.

'You must be Rose,' said Sally, as she strode down the long hallway towards our little band.

'Yes, that's me,' agreed mum.

141

Sally took mum by the hand, and began to lead her away, leaving Heather and me standing together at the end of the hallway. Mum followed Sally without question.

'I want you to tell me all about your very interesting life, Rose,' said Sally, 'and then I'll show you up to your room.'

Sally and mum disappeared through a white door at the other end of the corridor.

'There are some papers for you to sign,' said a young nurse who had suddenly joined us, 'as the next of kin.'

I nodded and signed the papers; I am sure I never even read them.

'Your mum is on the first floor in room six,' explained the nurse. 'You can bring her things up straight away.'

Heather followed the nurse up the sharp flight of stairs, and I went back to the car to retrieve mum's suitcase.

I had to ring the bell again to be re-admitted.

The nurse who opened the door smiled at me. 'Security,' she said.

'Room six?' I said.

'First floor, turn left,' she said, before disappearing into a small office and shutting the door behind her. I was left standing alone in the hallway. As I approached the stairs someone grabbed my hand. The grip was weak and cold. I looked up to see a very old lady, her cheeks badly tear-stained.

'Please!' she said, in a voice broken with age and emotion. '*Please!*'

'Now, now, Maud,' remonstrated a nurse, as she prised the old lady's hand from my wrist. 'Leave the nice man alone.'

Maud was led away through another door, sobbing as she went. I hauled my mum's suitcase up the stairs with my conscience in torment, and a heart as heavy as concrete. Room six was Charlie's old room, but his photograph had been removed from the wall outside. There was no trace of him anywhere, no evidence of his existence at all, except for threadbare Fred, who wandered past the room as I entered. Again he had a box of dominoes in his hand, and as he passed the room he glanced in. When he saw my mum and Heather sitting on the bed together he shook his head and moved on.

'This is very nice, indeed,' said mum, looking around. 'How long are we staying?'

'Just for a few days,' I said, feeling like Judas.

Heather began to unpack mum's suitcase and to put her clothes away into the wardrobe and the chest of drawers.

'I haven't brought my swimsuit,' said mum.

'We can get one tomorrow,' I lied.

Sally strolled into the room.

'Hello, Rose,' she said cheerily. 'Are you settling in all right?'

'I haven't brought my swimsuit, and I'd like to go to the beach,' said mum.

Sally took it all in her stride.

'Oh, Rose, it's much too cold for the beach today, we'll see what the weather's like tomorrow, alright?'

'I suppose it will have to be,' replied mum.

When mum was unpacked, Heather and I sat with her for a while. We didn't know how long we would be allowed to stay, and neither of us wanted to leave. Sally resolved the dilemma.

'Rose, Heather and Martin are coming downstairs with me now, there are some papers to sign. You wait here and make yourself comfortable. They'll come back and see you in a little while.'

I kissed mum goodbye. At least, *I* knew it was goodbye; she thought it was just a kiss.

Sally closed mum's door behind us, and we walked slowly down the upper landing towards the stairs.

'It's best you don't come back and see mum for a week or two,' said Sally. 'If you keep popping back in, she will never settle in properly, she'll keep thinking that you've come to take her home, and then she'll be upset. That's not fair to her, is it?'

We nodded in agreement that it wasn't fair.

'Come back and see us in a week or two when mum has settled in, and we can give you a progress report, okay?'

We nodded, shook hands with Sally, and left my mother still upstairs in Charlie's old room, thinking she was in a hotel on her holidays, and that she might be going to the beach tomorrow.

I wonder how long she sat on the bed waiting for us to come back.

16. Captain John

HEATHER AND I DROVE home from that place in silence. My mind was in turmoil: I felt as if I had just betrayed and abandoned my mother. What would my dad have made of my behaviour?

I was lost in this mental morass when Heather broke the spell.

'We won't leave it two weeks, no matter what that Sally says.'

I agreed at once.

'We'll go and see her next weekend, shall we?'

'Yes, that would be better.'

When Heather and I walked back into the house the silence was crashing. Bruno sat and looked at us. He greeted me, then Heather, then looked around. We both knew who he was looking for. I made a fuss of him that night, and took him out for a walk.

Later that evening, as the sun went down, we switched on the Christmas tree lights, purely out of habit. It was the middle of March.

Heather and I stood with our arms around each other just looking at the fairy lights, neither of us speaking. At last I broke the silence.

'I think it's time to take the Christmas tree down,' I said.

Heather nodded. That night she and I took down the eternal Christmas tree. When all its little lights were carefully stored away, and the bedraggled tree itself was broken down into sections and put back into its box, and the tinsel removed and bagged, the room looked so lonely and bare. I think I realised in that very moment that I couldn't live here any longer.

We were saying goodbye to Bruno, too. Someone once said that people come into your life for a reason or a season. When the reason for their visit ends, they leave; or if their season is over, then they move on, and so do you. Some people wander into our lives to support us in a time of crisis and then they fade out again. Others come to teach a lesson, and when the lesson is learned, they leave. I wonder if the same is true of animals? A few days later, Bruno's owner asked for him back. She was settled now, and, while she was very grateful to me for helping her out, she was now able to give the boy a home again. We arranged to meet the next day at a spot convenient for us both, and Bruno was handed over. It may be fanciful, but that dog was a great comfort to my mother when she needed one; he seemed to arrive at exactly the right time for her, and as soon as his services were no longer required he went home. I suppose mum arrived at the right time for Bruno, too. It's funny how things work out.

Heather and I passed the week by going out every night, either to the pub or for a meal. Neither of us really liked to stay in the house any more; it felt empty, lonely and cold, and it had been so long since we had spent an evening with just the two of us that we tried to make the most of it.

Towards the end of the week, she started to organise another suitcase full of stuff we could take to mum at the weekend.

'Shampoo and conditioner,' called Heather, from the list she had prepared.

'Check,' I said, and the shampoo and conditioner were tossed into the case on the bed.

'One large bath towel, one medium-sized towel, one hand towel, one facecloth.'

'Check.'

'One orange cardigan, one blue cardigan, one brown pleated skirt.'

'Check.'

We worked our way down a list that had been put together with military forethought and precision – Heather had done a much better job of imagining mum's requirements than I ever would have. When everything on the list was found to be present and correct, and the case was full, I slammed the lid shut.

'I hope she's been all right this week,' I said. 'On her own, I mean.'

'I hope so, too,' said Heather, 'but what happens if she hasn't been?'

'I know. I've been thinking about that. What if she hates it in there? We can't just take her home again, we'd all be back at square one.'

146

'We'd have to find her another home, and quick,' said Heather.

I shook my head. 'There wasn't anywhere else.'

On Sunday morning, we put mum's suitcase into the car and set off. I was a little apprehensive when I rang the old-fashioned bell this time. I had no way of preparing myself, no idea of what to expect.

Sally bustled into the hall to greet us again. 'Mum's settling in very well,' she said, cheerily. 'She's even made a new friend.'

I think both Heather and I must have breathed a loud sigh of relief. We went up the stairs again to room six, where I noticed a Polaroid snapshot of mum pinned to the wall. We opened the door. The room was empty. The bed had been remade, but the clothes we had put away when mum first arrived all seemed undisturbed. I wondered what she had been wearing all week. There was a very strong smell of urine; we traced it to a litter bin under the window, which contained a heavily soiled pair of mum's pants wrapped loosely in a polythene bag. Mum had been incontinent for some time now, and we had been buying disposable ones.

'I'll find mum and get rid of this,' I said to Heather, as I picked up the bag from inside the litter bin.

Together we went in search of my mother.

We found her wandering down one of the home's many corridors, hand-in-hand with an elderly male patient. He was taller than mum, had a good head of snow-white hair and a brown, suntanned face.

'Hello, Richard,' said mum, smiling broadly when she saw us, 'and hello, Wendy. I wondered if you would come and see me. This is Terry.'

Terry put out his hand and Heather and I shook it in turn. He was wearing his sweater inside out and back to front; the label was under his chin and the name 'John' was written in black ink across it. I looked down. His shoelaces were tied so that the bow was under the sole of the shoe.

'Storm's coming up,' announced Terry, or John. 'Going to be choppy.'

We nodded. It was a lovely spring day outside.

'So how have you been, mum?' I asked. 'How are you settling in?'

She broke into a huge smile at me, and then at Heather. Then she looked up with great affection at Terry. Then she looked back at me.

'I have something to tell you,' she said. 'I'm going to have a baby.'

Under normal circumstances, such an announcement made by someone's 80-year-old mother would probably be the cause of a certain amount of alarm. But I had been looking after her for nearly three years by this point, and wasn't so easily thrown.

'Jesus,' I said, as Heather laughed. 'You've only been here a week.'

'Terry and I are going to call it Martin, if it's a boy, and Peggy, if it's a girl,' announced mum. 'We're very happy, aren't we Terry?'

'Have to secure the hatches,' replied Terry.

We all nodded, as though we knew what he was talking about. Terry then let go of mum's hand and leaned against the corridor wall. I thought he was going to fall, and I sprang forward to catch him by the arm. A nearby nurse saw this and came over.

'Come on, Captain John,' she said. 'Leave Rose and her family to enjoy their visit. You can see Rose again later.'

The nurse began to guide Terry away from us. As they went the old man and the young nurse began to sway to the side, and Terry grabbed the wall again.

'Oh, it's a bit choppy today, Captain,' remarked the young nurse.

'Storm's coming,' remarked Terry, as they wandered away.

Another nurse, who had been standing with her colleague had witnessed this, and came over to us.

'Take no notice of Captain John,' she said. 'He's one of our longer-term residents.'

'So he's not Terry?' I said, looking at mum.

'No, it's John,' replied the nurse. 'He was in the Royal Navy for years. We call him Captain John. He thinks he lives on a boat.'

We all watched Captain John and the young nurse disappear away down the corridor together, he grabbing the wall again as he walked and the imaginary deck rolled under him.

The nurse smiled at me. 'The sea's rough today,' she said, and moved away.

'Isn't he lovely?' said mum, with a romantic sigh when they had turned the corner at the end of the corridor, and were now out of sight.

'His name's John, not Terry,' said Heather.

'I know, Wendy,' said mum. 'I get confused.'

'Well, I'm glad you've made a new friend,' I said.

Mum smiled at me. 'Terry brings me such nice presents, Richard.'

'That's nice,' I said, and the three of us wandered back to her room.

We sat mum on the bed and unpacked her case. We hung up the new clothes we had brought for her, and went through the list of the things we had brought the first time. There were a lot of items missing. Skirts and blouses that had belonged to mum were no longer in her room, and in their place we found some items that were not hers.

'It's very difficult to keep track of who owns what,' explained a nurse whom I had called into the room to ask her about this.

'But you asked us to mark all her clothes with her name before she came in,' replied Heather. 'We've done that, and there are still things missing.'

'But they wander in and out of each other's rooms all the time,' replied the nurse. 'Sometimes they just take things and forget to bring them back. Of course some of the missing items could be in the laundry.'

'Can we see the laundry?' asked Heather.

'It's closed today,' said the nurse, quickly – a little too quickly, I thought.

Later we were to discover why we were not allowed to see the laundry.

'Are you getting enough to eat, mum?' I asked.

'Oh yes, there's plenty to eat,' replied mum. 'Are the band coming to see me?'

Heather and I looked at each other. 'Er… They've gone home,' I said.

Mum nodded. 'She's come here with me.'

'Who has?' asked Heather.

Mum nodded her head slowly towards the radiator in her bedroom.

'Is the little girl still stuck in there?' I asked.

Mum nodded.

Captain John walked in. 'I've brought you a present, Rose,' he said.

He handed mum a long, black, plastic box, designed to store 10 cassette tapes in a row. The box, which was empty, had lost its lid and was split down one side. It looked like someone had stood on it.

Tears sprang into mum's eyes. 'Oh, Terry,' she said, kissing his cheek. 'It's absolutely beautiful. Thank you very much.'

Mum ran her fingers lovingly down the length of the broken box.

Captain John looked directly at me. 'Wind's freshening.'

I nodded and smiled.

'Terry brings me beautiful presents, doesn't he?' said mum.

'It's lovely,' agreed Heather.

'I want you to arrange a priest to come here and marry me and Terry,' said mum. 'We're going to have a baby.'

'I'll see what I can do,' I replied.

We bade farewell to mum and Captain John and the nurses, and made our way out.

* * * * *

There is a sense of progressive hopelessness surrounding dementia that I believe not even cancer can rival.

We visited mum every week for the next 18 months, on each occasion bringing her clothes from home and boxes of chocolates. On one particular visit we opened her wardrobe door to find the compartment completely empty.

'Where are all your clothes?' I asked.

'I don't know, ask Peggy,' came the familiar reply.

The nurse looked very sheepish when we questioned her about this. 'They might be in the laundry,' she ventured.

'Can we go to the laundry?' asked Heather.

'I think it's closed today,' the nurse replied.

'It's always closed when we want to see it,' replied Heather. 'Can we speak to Sally?'

'I think it's her day off,' said the nurse, looking down at the floor.

'Okay, thank you,' I said, and the nurse left.

'I'm going to get to the bottom of this,' said Heather. 'You wait here with mum.'

She went in search of some answers.

Mum and I sat on the bed together in silence. When every conversation you have with someone is filled with fantasy and delusion, and finding the truth is as tricky as herding cats, sooner or later you run out of things to say.

'How is the little girl in the radiator these days?' I asked, lamely. It was the only thing I could think of to say.

Mum shook her head sadly. 'She's all right, I suppose,' she replied, looking at the radiator in the room.

'She's still in there then?' I asked.

'I think they'll never let her out now,' replied mum softly. 'They've all forgotten about her.'

I put my arm around mum's shoulder.

'I want you to write a letter for me,' announced mum, changing the subject.

'Okay, what's it about?' I asked.

'I want you to complain to the train company. After what they did to us something needs to be done.'

I frowned. 'What happened?'

'The bloody train broke down, and we all had to walk back here from Gloucester. And me in my underwear. It's not right to treat old people like that.'

'What were you all doing in Gloucester?' I asked. It's really hard not to get sucked in.

'We went to Princess Diana's wedding, of course,' said mum. 'Terry was invited because he's such an important person, and he took all of us with him.'

'Oh, of course,' I agreed.

Alzheimer's is like a religion: it requires neither reason nor logic, only belief. It would have been absolutely pointless to mention that Princess Diana's wedding had been years ago, in London and not Gloucester, that it was unlikely that Captain John would have been invited to the ceremony anyway, and that the train company, for all their faults, would be equally unlikely to strand a bunch of elderly commuters (all in their underwear) miles from home. All of that was beside the point.

Incidentally, a quick investigation with the nurses solved this one easily. In the morning several of the residents had gathered in the television lounge to watch a documentary on the Royal family, which had included footage of Lady Diana Spencer's marriage to Prince Charles. This programme had been followed by an episode of *Thomas the Tank Engine*. In mum's mind, the storylines of the two programmes had simply merged together into one real-life episode. Why she had been in her underwear at the time was anyone's guess, though.

She gave me a pen and some paper, and waited while I wrote the letter. When I had finished she made me read it back to her. She seemed quite satisfied with the result.

To Whom This May Concern,

I am writing on behalf of my mother and a number of other elderly residents, currently residing at_____, who have been shamefully treated by your company, and who were left in a state of danger and distress when you saw fit to turf them all off a train in Gloucester, clad in nothing but their underwear. They all had to walk back to Coventry, some 50 miles, some with no shoes, and others with no knickers or teeth.

I look forward to your comments and your proposals for compensation.

Yours faithfully,

Martin Slevin.

Mum liked the last bit about compensation.

'That's a very good letter,' she said. 'That should teach them a lesson.'

Heather came back into the bedroom.

'That laundry down there is an absolute disgrace,' she announced. 'It's no wonder they didn't want us to see it.' She joined us on the edge of the bed. 'There's one young lad down there on his own, he hardly speaks any English, and hasn't got a clue what he's doing. He's boil-washing everything. All the coloureds and whites together, all the woollens and cottons and silks, all together. All your mum's woollen jumpers have shrunk to half their size, she can't wear any of them. Her nice pleated skirts have all been boiled to death. All her clothes are ruined. We need to see the manager... Where's Sally?'

Sally wasn't on duty, but Heather had determined to do something about the ruined clothes. When we got home we started to make a list of what had been destroyed.

Next day at work, I bought a box of chocolates and sent them to mum with a letter.

Dear Rose,

I was so sorry to hear about your misadventure with Thomas in Gloucester. This was very unfortunate, and I promise it will never happen again.

Please accept these chocolates which you can share with your friends, by way of an apology.

Yours sincerely,

The Fat Controller.

17. A Formal Complaint

WE WENT BACK to the home the next day, and took with us the original inventory of mum's clothes. We searched her room, searched other people's rooms, and searched the laundry trying to locate her stuff. When we put the pile together, we checked it off against the original list, and we were astonished. She'd only been in this home for three months or so. In that time, the clothes they had lost would cost – at a conservative estimate – £1,300 to replace.

I decided to write a letter to Sally – a serious one, this time.

Dear Sally,

I am astonished to discover that almost the entire contents of my mother's wardrobe has either been lost or destroyed by the incompetence of your laundry service. A service consisting of, I understand, one non-English speaking, under-age, foreign national with no training.

I enclose a list of the damage and loss, and look forward to hearing from you in due course.

CLOTHES MISSING FROM ORIGINAL INVENTORY

22 pairs of knickers (£88.00), 1 brown handbag (£25.00), All toiletries (£25.00), 5 bras (£75.00), 1 white nightdress (£10.00), 1 floral nightdress (£10.00), 1 pair of light grey trousers (£20.00), 1 pair of dark grey trousers (£20.00), 3 pairs of towelling socks (£6.99), 2 face flannels (£5.00), 3 bath towels (£36.00), 1 lemon blouse (£15.00), 1 dark purple blouse (£24.99), 1 beige skirt (Berkatex, box-pleated at front) (£37.99), 2 hand towels (£14.00), 1 pair pyjamas (£10.00), 1 light green skirt (Berkatex, box-pleated at front) (£37.99), 1 cream short-sleeved blouse (£10.00), 1 black velour skirt (£20.00), 1 brown velour skirt (£20.00), 1 pink long-sleeved cardigan (£25.00), 1 lilac short-sleeved jumper (£20.00), 1 pair of fur lined winter boots (£55.99), 1 blue frilled nightdress (£10.00), 3 white plain nightdresses (£30.00), 1 plain v-neck t-shirt (£8.00), 1 pink v-neck with white collar t-shirt (£10.00), 3 pairs of cotton socks, blue, purple and white (£5.99), 1 pink blouse (£15.00), 1 pair of black trousers (£20.00), 1 dark red tie-up blouse (£24.99)

CLOTHING RUINED IN THE LAUNDRY
13 skirts (£390.00), 1 purple blouse (£28.99), 1 pink jumper (£20.00), 1 green blouse (£20.00), 1 sky blue jumper (£25.00), 1 blue all-in-one jumper (£25.00), 1 green cardigan (£24.99), 1 lemon blouse (£15.00), 1 pyjama top (£10.00), 1 cream silk pair of shorts (£5.00), 1 plain lilac top (£5.00), 1 large pink woollen jumper (£15.00)

I also notice that you have recently sent me a bill for £1,500 in respect of accommodation charges at your establishment; obviously that will not now be paid until the matter at hand is settled amicably.

Yours faithfully,
MARTIN SLEVIN

Sally never replied. I did, however, receive another bill for £1,500 for mum's stay, with no reference at all to my complaint.

There exists in the UK a committee which was set up to oversee care homes, to ensure they work to a well-defined standard and to deal independently with complaints like mine. I wrote to the committee describing my grievances, and enclosing a copy of the above letter to Sally. The committee eventually replied to me.

Dear Mr Slevin,

After an extensive investigation at the _____ nursing home, in which we asked Mrs Sally _____ to look into your claims, she assures us that her staff are fully trained, and that all reasonable precautions were taken for the maintenance of your mother's clothes; however you must understand that mistakes do happen, and if that has been the case here, then we apologise. We were informed by Mrs Sally _____ that a member of staff spent a considerable amount of time conducting a thorough search and found the majority of the missing items in Mrs Slevin's room.

We trust that this brings the matter to an end, and look forward to you resuming good relations with the home you have chosen for your mother's residence.

Faithfully,

I couldn't believe that this so-called professional body, who were supposed to oversee such poor nursing homes, did not even bother to visit the place to investigate my complaint. Instead, they asked the manageress of the home to investigate herself on their behalf and, unsurprisingly, she found nothing to be amiss.

I contacted the social worker and lodged a formal complaint with her, but I was so disenchanted with the whole process that I held out no optimism for a satisfactory conclusion from her department either.

The next week Heather and I visited the home, packed mum's suitcase with the rags she had left, and walked out with her. One of the nurses started to cry as we left.

'I'm so sorry about this,' she whispered to me, as we walked mum down the corridor, 'but there's nothing we can do. We can't say anything or we'll lose our jobs.'

I nodded to her. I did understand her position – and many of the individual nurses had been kindness itself – but if no-one ever takes a stand in matters like these, if no-one is prepared to defend these unfortunate souls who cannot defend themselves, then the irresponsible and incompetent people who run such places are never made to pay.

Captain John waved to mum as we walked towards the door. I felt so sorry for taking her away from her new friend, but I felt I had no choice.

'Where are we going?' she asked, as we walked back to the car.

'We're going to another hotel, mum,' I lied.

'Ooh, you two really do spoil me,' she said. 'I've never had such lovely, long holidays!'

I replied to the committee as a last resort, but I held no hope for any real satisfaction:

Dear _____,

I am in receipt of your letter dated 19th July, and find myself lost for words quite frankly!

You state that on your behalf Mrs Sally _____ investigated my complaint!! You have therefore allowed one of this home's staff to investigate themselves. If they are to do this what is the point in contacting an independent commission such as yourselves?

The reply I received was full of inconsistencies, untruths and misleading statements, and in no way am I either happy or satisfied with the way you have handled this matter.

To take issue with only one point in your letter as an example:

'A member of staff spent a considerable amount of time conducting a thorough search and found the majority of the missing items in Mrs Slevin's room.'

This is simply not the case, and you will see by the itemised list attached that over 80% of the clothes my mother arrived with were either lost or destroyed during her short stay there. In fact the state of her clothes was so bad that several of the home's own staff were in tears and repeatedly apologised to us when we went to pick up Mrs Slevin, the day we moved her away from the home.

We have had to replace the underwear and toiletries and nightwear already. Some of the items listed were new which we removed the labels from the day she was settled into the home. The total cost of replacements is £1,319.91, which does not include the large pile of clothes which we left at the home, as they were unfit to wear, due to rips, shrinkage, tears and discolouring due to poor laundry.

In the event of this I do not feel that I owe them anything, and will not be settling the £1,500 bill they have the cheek to keep sending me.

Faithfully,

Martin Slevin.

We drove home, mum happily enjoying the view, me wondering what the hell I was going to do now. As it happened, the social worker rang within a couple of hours.

'I've got you a place at a new home,' she said. 'Charnwood House. It's much nicer. Can you pop over to see it, do you think?'

We said we could.

Maybe I was just being suspicious and cynical, but it seemed to me that this new place had quickly become available when I started to cause a disturbance in the 'system'; when I had first enquired, and was not being disruptive, I was told more or less to take it or leave what was offered. The more I came to deal with the Social Services over the years, the more I came to the unshakeable conclusion that you get nowhere by being civilised and polite. The more you bang your fist on the table and make demands and issue threats, the more likely you are to get what you want. It shouldn't be like that, but unfortunately it is; and if you ever find yourself in the position of being a carer for a member of your family with dementia, and you have to deal with Social Services, then be prepared to speak out loudly. You will need to be a warrior on their behalf, their champion at arms, you will need to be prepared to fight their battles for them, and there will be no shortage of bureaucratic dragons for you to slay.

18. Second Home

WE LOCKED THE DOOR and set off straight away for Charnwood House. As we pulled into the car park and stopped, I was struck by its neatly-clipped lawns and flower beds. The building was a solid, one-storey affair, too; there was no issue of dangerous stairways for the visiting relative to consider.

'This looks nice,' said Heather.

We crossed the asphalt and rang the bell to the main reception. A voice came through on the intercom a couple of seconds later.

'Can I help you?'

'We've come to look around,' I said, and the front door clicked softly open.

We entered a spacious hallway and were met by a middle-aged lady with a ready smile and kind eyes.

'Welcome to Charnwood House,' she said, shaking our hands. 'Let me show you around.'

Our guide ushered us through a set of coded security doors into an open and expansive seating area, which was fresh-smelling and tidy. A few elderly residents were dotted here and there; mostly, they were sound asleep. A fairly forgettable but pleasant melody was playing quietly over the speaker system.

'We hold our bingo sessions and our sing-songs in here,' she said. 'As you can see, it's very light and spacious... There's a nice atmosphere, don't you think?'

There was: this place was the opposite of mum's former home. Where that had been dark and depressing, this was light and cheerful. Where that had been a rabbit warren of narrow, cold corridors and steep, winding staircases, this was a giant, open-planned bungalow. Where that had been an old house converted to lock in elderly patients with dementia, this was a purpose-built facility for their comfort and welfare. Heather and I knew then we had made the right decision in moving mum. I knew she would love it here.

'This is another lounge, which we also use as the dining room,' said our host, as we wandered down the large central corridor. 'We have two spare rooms... Let me show them to you.'

The bedrooms, like the rest of the building, were nicely painted, bright and comfortable. They looked more like the cabins on a cruise ship than the bedrooms of a care home. Captain John would have been right at home here. We carried on, and passed a hairdressing salon.

'Each Wednesday a very good ladies' hairdresser works in there,' said our guide, 'so your mother can have her hair done. Once a month we have a visiting chiropodist and a dentist.'

I thought about the non-existent facilities of mum's previous home; how could they be so different?

'What do you think?' asked our guide. 'Would she be comfortable here?'

'Absolutely,' replied Heather.

'Definitely,' said I, and the deal was done.

* * * * *

We installed mum the following day.

'This is a beautiful hotel,' she observed, looking around. 'How on earth can we afford to stay here?'

'Let me worry about that,' I replied.

'I'll ask them if I can have breakfast in bed tomorrow morning,' whispered mum, as we showed her to her new room. It had a lovely view over a vast flowerbed and rose garden. 'Are you *sure* we can afford to stay here?' she asked again, looking out of the window. 'It must cost a fortune.'

'This is your home now, mum,' replied Heather. 'Better than the last place, isn't it?'

Mum nodded. 'I didn't like that other place,' she said.

Heather and I looked at each other.

'I hope she's nice,' said mum, pointing to the other single bed in the room.

'That bed's not used,' I said. 'I've already asked about it. It's just a spare bed they have put in here. You have this room all to yourself.'

'I hope she isn't going to snore all night, and keep me awake,' said mum, 'or I'll have to tell her.'

'There won't *be* anyone in that bed,' I said. 'There's just you in here.'

'And if she starts talking in her sleep, I'll give her such a dig in the ribs!' announced mum.

From her very first day at Charnwood House to her last, mum continued to believe she was staying in a top-class hotel. She thought all the nursing staff were waiters and waitresses, and she used to tell the other 'guests' that I had won the lottery, and was keeping her in luxury. It was a delusion I did not contradict.

We put what was left of mum's clothes into her wardrobe, and we started to settle her in. Then there was a knock on the door.

'I would like to take mum around and introduce her to everyone,' said a young nurse. 'Let's see if we can make her some new friends.'

Heather and I smiled, and mum took the nurse's hand like a child, and the two of them went off together.

'I can rest easier, knowing she's being looked after in here,' I said to Heather.

'We should bring down some photographs and personal ornaments, that sort of thing, to put in her room,' remarked Heather. 'It will make the place more personal to her.'

'We need to buy her some more clothes too,' I said.

Heather nodded. 'Let's go shopping.'

We spent a small fortune replacing as many as we could of the items which had either been lost or ruined in the previous home. We took the clothes and toiletries back to the bungalow with us so we could write mum's name on all the labels before giving them to her. We decided to give her a settling-in week, as before, and so the following weekend we paid mum her first visit in her new home.

'I want you to write me a letter,' announced mum, the moment we arrived.

Here we go again, I thought.

'Every morning they come in and wake us up for breakfast. I always get up straight away, but that poor woman always wants a lie in.' She pointed to the other bed in her room.

'Yes,' I said.

'Well,' mum went on indignantly, 'because she won't get up when they call her, they come in and drag her out of bed by her feet!' Heather and I tried not to laugh. 'They shouldn't be dragging old people out of bed like that in the morning, should they?'

We agreed that they really shouldn't.

Mum went to her bedside table and brought back a sheet of plain paper and a pen. I knew she would want me to write the letter there and then. I composed the complaint, supervised the whole time by mum looking over my shoulder.

'What's her name?' I asked.

'I don't know,' replied mum. 'She never speaks to me.'

Dear Sir or Madam,

I am writing to complain about the way Mrs Slevin's room-mate is dragged out of her bed by her feet every morning. Obviously this is contrary to the Health & Safety at Work Act, as this lady could easily bump her head when she hits the floor. This is distressing to Mrs Slevin, and we would request that you get the lady up in some other way.

Faithfully,

Martin Slevin.

'That's a very good letter,' announced mum when we were finished. 'You have to stick up for your friends, you know.'

'How are you settling in?' asked Heather.

'The food is lovely,' replied mum, enthusiastically, 'but I'd expect no less from such a swanky hotel.'

'I'm glad you like it here,' I said.

'Why wouldn't I like it?' asked mum. 'The waiters are very friendly and the service is always first class.'

'We've brought you some cream cakes,' said Heather. We had stopped at a baker's on the way and had bought a box of five various fancies.

'We can have one each and there will be two over, maybe your mum can give the other two to some friends,' Heather had said.

'Oh, that's wonderful, Wendy!' exclaimed mum. 'Let's have them now.'

She opened the box and took out a cream cake which she devoured in about two gulps. After I had wiped the cream off her face, she chose another.

'I've accepted Frank's proposal of marriage,' she said in a matter-of-fact way, between bites of a chocolate éclair. 'At my time of life, I have to think about the future, don't I?'

'I suppose you do,' agreed Heather.

'Who's Frank?' I said.

'My fiancée, of course!' replied mum, giving me a slightly pitying look and selecting a huge custard slice.

'You've met Frank in here, then?' asked Heather.

Mum nodded vigorously. Her mouth was full of pastry and cold custard. 'He's a fighter pilot with the Royal Air Force,' she said, proudly. 'We're going to live on a fighter base when we're married.'

'That's nice, mum,' I replied.

'I want you to arrange for a priest to come and do the service,' said mum. 'When can you get him here?'

'Leave it with me,' I sighed. 'I'll sort it out tomorrow.'

'Quick as you can, Richard. I don't want to look too pregnant when I go down the aisle,' said mum, taking the fourth cake from the box.

'But you've only just met this man, Frank, mum,' I said, and immediately regretted trying to inject some logic into the proceedings.

'What are you talking about?' asked mum. 'We've known each other since school. We've been engaged for years! No, it's high time we did the decent thing and made it all official. Besides,' she whispered, taking the fifth and final cake from the box, 'people are starting to talk.'

We showed mum the new clothes we had bought her, and hung them up in her wardrobe.

'They're beautiful!' she said. 'But you shouldn't spend so much money on me.'

'You have to have something to wear,' I replied.

'Well, confidentially,' she whispered, 'I have noticed that some of the guests here don't really dress that well. No-one seems to dress up any more these days, even when staying at a top hotel like this one. There are no standards any more.'

I nodded. That was something both Heather and I had noticed since we first started to visit care homes. Most of the patients of such places did seem to be dressed very poorly. I suppose there's some truth in what the nurse at the previous home had said – because the patients are in and out of each other's rooms all the time, borrowing things and never returning them, their relatives take the view that it isn't worth providing decent clothes. Given that most dementia patients couldn't care less how they look, anyway, is there any point in keeping up appearances?

'Well, you look very nice, anyway, Rose,' said Heather diplomatically.

'Thank you, Wendy,' replied mum. 'With Richard having such an important job, I think I owe it to him to look my best.'

'What important job have I got?' I asked.

'You know, with the animal training, and the bullfighting, and all that,' mum said, nodding at me conspiratorially.

'Bullfighting?' said Heather.

'Yes, you know, he does bullfighting for Coventry City Council. It's a very important job. Everyone knows that. Don't they, Richard?'

I just nodded.

'Someone has to keep all them mad cows under control,' observed mum, 'or the place would be overrun with… with… '

'Mad cows?' I ventured.

'Exactly!' agreed mum.

'Have you made any more friends?' asked Heather. 'Apart from Frank, I mean.'

When talking to dementia patients you quickly fall into the habit of regularly changing the subject before your brain starts to melt.

'Oh yes!' exclaimed mum. 'People are so friendly here. Apart from Mrs Whatshername, who's a right bitch. And the other little sneak. She comes in here and steals all my sweets, so now I hide them.'

'That's a good idea,' I said.

'What friends have you got then?' pursued Heather.

'I have plenty. There's old Mrs Fatbelly, she's very nice. She tells me things about the other guests. Do you know what she told me the other day?'

'No.' I said. I couldn't even begin to guess.

'She said that yer woman…' Mum jerked her head in the general direction of the door. 'Yer woman murdered all of her husbands for their insurance money. Isn't that a horrible thing to do? There ought to be a law against that!'

'There *is* a law against it, mum.'

'Well, she's done away with three of them,' she whispered. Then she leant in closer. 'But she's really very nice when you get to know her.'

19. The Dilemma Of The Talking Cat

HEATHER HAD BEEN living at mum's bungalow with me and trying to sell her own house. As neither of us really wanted to live at the bungalow any more, we decided to look for a place of our own – somewhere we could both make a fresh start.

We began house-hunting in earnest, and in the February of the following year we found a house that we both liked in Nuneaton, a small town a few miles north of Coventry. Heather's place had been sold in the meantime, and we bought the new home and moved in. Mum's bungalow was put up for sale, and an era for both Heather and myself came to an end.

Heather's ex-husband had owned a pair of cats, Smokey and Sandy, and they had been left with her when the marriage broke up. Heather had also taken on a couple of other moggies – Sprite and Tabitha – when her daughters had left home. Finally, my own daughter Rebecca had owned Barney, and he had wound up staying with me when Wendy and I had split up. To cut a long story short, when Heather and I moved to Nuneaton, we somehow took five cats with us. Cats are like that.

Sandy was a ginger tom who had been the runt of his litter; Heather and her family had nursed him back to health with TLC and many tender words whispered into his pointy little ears and, as a result, Sandy had become so responsive to a human voice that whenever anyone spoke to him he answered them back. One afternoon, I found myself in the front garden of the new house digging holes for Heather to pop plants into. The local infant school was emptying out, and gangs of small children were filing past on their way home. As Heather and I were chatting, Sandy was joining in with the conversation, as he invariably did, and I suddenly noticed that a small group of girls, around six years of age, had stopped behind me, and were listening. I thought I would have a bit of fun with them, and carried on talking, not to Heather, but to Sandy instead.

'So, Sandy, what did you say to that?' I asked.

'Meow, meow, meow.'

'Really? So what happened then?'

'Meow, meow, meow,' explained Sandy.

There was an excited mutter behind me. This was fun.

'No! You don't say... And did you fix the problem?'

'Meow, meow, meow,' replied Sandy.

'Well, I hope they were grateful to you,' I said, nodding at the cat.

And so it went on, me saying any old rubbish, and Sandy meowing perfectly on cue, as though answering me. Within a few minutes, there were gasps of excitement from the little group, who dispersed when their mothers arrived to take them home.

I thought no more about it, until the next Monday afternoon when there was a knock on the door. A pretty young woman stood there, hand-in-hand with one of the girls I recognised from the group who had listened to Sandy and me.

'I'm terribly sorry to bother you,' began the young woman, 'but all I've heard all weekend is, "When can we see the talking cat?" Just for the sake of peace, I thought I would knock the door, I hope you don't mind.'

'Sure,' I said, and invited them in. They stood in the kitchen, and I put Sandy on a chair.

'Sandy,' I said. 'This young lady has come to see you, isn't that nice?'

'Meow, meow, meow.'

Gasps from the little girl.

'Sandy says thank you very much... He doesn't get many visitors.'

'Meow, meow, meow.'

'He says you're a very nice little girl, and he hopes you always do as your mummy tells you.'

The young mum laughed, and the little girl was enthralled. Sandy continued to chatter away until he got bored with the game and ran off, but by then the little girl was more than ever convinced that we had a fantastic talking cat in our house. I could imagine the conversation in the school playground the following morning.

It wasn't until about a week later, when I was visiting mum, that something suddenly dawned upon me. We had been talking about the little girl in the radiator, and once again I had been going along with it.

'She tells me that people don't really listen to her stories any more,' said mum, looking wistfully at the radiator.

'Is that so?' I replied. 'Why does she think that?'

Then it hit me — that I was playing a game like that I'd played with the kids the week before. Then I'd had Sandy as a stooge, and the children — their immature intellects too young to spot the trick — had been easily duped. I was doing the same thing with mum. I was enforcing and supporting her delusion by playing along with it and she — her mind having regressed to its childhood capacity — was too infected with her Alzheimer's to spot the trick.

This is the dilemma of the talking cat, as I call it. Is it morally right to go along with your patient's delusions, just for the sake of a peaceful life? Or is it better to challenge whenever they arise, so that you are constantly dragging them back into your reality, and thereby upsetting and perhaps even frightening them, by being more concerned with your truth than their happiness?

Everyone who takes on the heavy burden of caring for a loved one like this will face this dilemma, sooner or later. They may try the second route instinctively first; it is when a challenge causes conflict to arise within the relationship — don't forget, the delusion is the patient's reality — that the carer may think twice.

The trouble is that, especially early in the evolution of a relative's condition, it upsets us to hear what is, objectively, nonsense talked by a person about whom we care so much — a person who would never have dreamt of saying such things before. We want the disease to go away, and our loved one to return to the stable mental state of old, when all was well. We want the person we remember returned to us; their delusions sharply remind us that this can never happen. I think the Alzheimer's fantasy is almost an attack on our own memories, an assault on our own love, and an evil that needs to be fought and resisted.

Not long after mum moved to her second home, I challenged the validity of the little girl in the radiator. I'm not sure why – I think it was done instinctively, without any serious thought at all.

'I don't know why you keep going on about that stupid girl inside the radiator,' I remember saying. 'There can be no such thing.'

It was a brutal rebuttal, delivered with the mighty strength of pure ignorance.

Mum had looked hurt, shocked, and horrified all at once. She closed down, refused to speak again, and distanced herself so quickly from me that I was left sitting there feeling as though I had let a bomb go off. I tried to build a bridge straight away, but made it out of paper as I tried to reinforce my point by arguing the logic of it. I could not have handled it any more incompetently if I had planned to do so.

'Surely you must realise no little girl could possibly live in there?' I said, pointing to the slim radiator on the wall.

Mum turned her head away, looked out of the window and did not reply. She was now somewhere else entirely, and all contact with her was lost.

'Mum, just think about it logically for a moment,' I persisted.

When you find yourself standing in a massive hole, it's wise to stop digging. Mum moved her head further away from my direction, and folded her arms. She reminded me of a child refusing point-blank to eat her dinner. Even I knew then that my position was hopeless. I changed the subject.

'Do you want a chocolate?' I asked, holding out a freshly-opened box. Mum had always loved her sweets and chocolates, and even the ravages of her mental condition had been unable to take that away from her. I could usually win her over with confectionery. She simply shook her head in silence. All hope of reconnecting for the time being now really was lost.

'I'd better go then,' I said.

I leaned over and kissed her. 'I'll see you next time,' I said, and left.

I never challenged her again. We all have our own private delusions, anyway; it's just that Alzheimer's patients have them to a marked degree. And to point out the obvious to her could solve nothing; it would never change her mind and instead would only create conflict, and widen the gap between us. All my little pet theories about handling mum, and Alzheimer's patients in general, were born like this, out of trial and error; no-one had written a book for me, and I often thought later that life would have been so much simpler if they had. The dilemma of the talking cat, despite its quirky name, is a real problem that all carers eventually have to face. How you deal with it… well, you make up your own mind.

* * * * *

I visited mum every week; usually at the weekends, but if I could manage it I would often drop in during the week as well. I decided that I would visit her sooner rather than later this time to try to repair some of the damage I had done to our relationship by challenging the concept of the little girl in the radiator. I had been thinking about the episode constantly, and had decided it was futile to challenge the logic of her fantasies. It solved nothing; it would not change her mind and could only widen the gap between us.

I visited her on the following Wednesday afternoon, my mind made up that I would act as if the previous visit had never happened; I would not apologise for it, nor allude to it in any way. My hope was that, because her short-term memory was so fragile, if I did not remind her of it she might not recall it either.

'Hi, mum!' I said cheerily. 'How are you doing?'

'Oh, Richard!' she exclaimed, her face breaking into a huge smile. 'How lovely to see you.'

All was well.

It was a little awkward at first, as I could never be completely sure whether or not she remembered the details of previous visits. If she had, then she made a very good job of pretending, and it was my guess that the events of only a few days ago were just so much of her forgotten history now; they may as well have happened a thousand years before.

Mum glanced periodically at the small, white enamel radiator on her bedroom wall. I thought I should broach the subject that stood between us, and tackled it head-on, but in a different way this time.

'Have you been talking to the little girl in there again?' I asked.

Mum nodded her head vigorously. 'She talks to me all the time,' she said.

'How is she doing today?' I asked.

'She's not so sad today,' replied mum.

Her face had softened into a gentle look and was graced by an easy smile. The difference between the way she looked now, and the face she had offered to me at the time of my last visit was so marked that they could have belonged to two completely different people.

'What do you two find to talk about all day?' I asked.

'We talk about all sorts of things,' replied mum, warming to her favourite subject. 'We chat all the time. She understands lots of things, you know. Grown-ups don't always realise how much children actually do know. They don't miss a trick!'

'Do you ever hear her say things that upset you?'

'Never!' Mum seemed very determined on this point. 'When she tells me things I know that they're true, so they don't upset me even if I don't like what she says sometimes.'

'What has she said that you didn't like, mum?'

Mum seemed to be contemplating the question for a moment.

'She whispers things to me sometimes, when it's dark, late at night and there are just the two of us in the room, and when no-one else can hear us.'

'What did she say to you that you didn't like though?'

'She said that everyone on the outside thinks that we're all mad in here, and we're not. Well, I'm not anyway.'

'No, of course you're not mad, and people on the outside don't think that you are, anyway,' I said.

'Then why would she say such a thing?' asked mum. 'If it wasn't true?'

'Maybe she was just playing a joke on you.'

'Yes, that must be it,' replied mum, nodding in agreement.

She fell into a thoughtful silence, her mind fully engaged with thoughts of her little friend.

There was a soft knock on the door. A young nurse in a smart blue uniform popped her head around the door.

'Rose, we're starting to serve our evening meal now, in the lounge,' she said. 'Would you like to have yours in your room, or are you going to join the others?'

'No, I'll come down,' replied mum.

The nurse closed the bedroom door quietly behind her.

'I have to go for my supper now,' said mum. 'Will you come down and have a bite with us?'

'No, I'd better be going.' I said.

'Come and meet my friends, then,' said mum.

We left her room arm-in-arm, and walked the short distance to the TV lounge where supper was being served.

20. Mum's Little Gang

AS MUM BECAME more and more a part of the Charnwood House furniture, she seemed to gather about her a large circle of intimates, some of whom drifted away as others joined the little band. There was a hard-core membership of around half-a-dozen who sat with mum constantly, and Heather and I referred to them as 'Mum's Little Gang'.

Because the symptoms of Alzheimer's are very individual to the sufferer, each member of Mum's Little Gang had their own peculiarities and idiosyncrasies. At times, these would interact well with the personalities of the other members; at times, they would make a crashing contrast.

I remember on one occasion, Heather and I had come to visit mum, and the gang were all there in the lounge together.

'You two can fuck off!' shouted one of the ladies as we entered.

The rest of the ladies rolled their eyes and tutted their disapproval.

'This is Richard and Wendy,' announced mum, introducing us to everyone. 'My brother and my son's wife.'

'Hello Dick!' shouted another of the gang, an ancient specimen of womanhood sitting in the corner. 'How's your dick?' And then she began to shriek with laughter. 'How's your dick, Dick?'

The others raised their eyes to the ceiling and they all tutted again.

'Pay no attention to her,' suggested mum. 'She's very common.'

One of mum's pals got out of her chair and made her way unsteadily around the furniture to where we were standing.

'You mustn't be upset by that old witch,' whispered this lady. 'She's a bit gone in the head, so you have to make allowances.'

'We will, don't worry,' replied Heather.

'I mean, she's not all there,' continued the lady, waving her index finger in circles next to her ear and raising her eyes, in the classic playground sign for 'loopy'. 'A bit gone in the head, she is.'

'I understand,' I said.

'I mean, she doesn't really know what she's saying most of the time,' continued the lady.

'Yes, we understand,' I assured her.

'A bit gone in the head she is,' repeated the lady again, and started to wave her finger around in circles next to her ear again.

'Sit down, Joyce,' said mum, catching this lady by the sleeve. 'They don't want to be hearing all that.'

'I was just saying she's a bit gone in the head,' remarked Joyce, and away went her finger again.

'Fuck off and sit down, you stupid cow!' shouted the lady who had first greeted us.

Joyce rolled her eyes towards the ceiling, and then went back to her chair.

One of the gang had a collection of children's wind-up toys on the table. She was hunched over the table winding up each toy and then letting it go. A little red duck waddled across the table.

'Weeeee!' shouted the lady. 'Look at that!' and she giggled so loudly that many of the others laughed as well.

Then the lady with the toys wound up a small plastic dog and let it go.

'Weeeee!' she shouted again, laughing as the dog ran across the table.

'Fuck off with them stupid toys!' shouted the first lady again.

Joyce struggled up and came back round to us. 'Don't mind her with those toys, she's a bit gone in the head, she is.'

'Oh, Joyce!' shouted someone else. 'Sit down!'

'I'm having a chat with Dick!' shouted back Joyce. 'I'm telling him something very important!'

'How's your dick, Dick?' screamed the ancient lady again, and then roared with laughter.

'Fuck off with that fucking dick, Dick!' bawled the first one.

There was another lady at the table who had done nothing but whistle since we had arrived. She whistled the same four notes over and over, without ever stopping for breath. We later found out that this lady rarely spoke a word to anyone, even when asked a direct question; all she ever did was whistle the same four notes in the same order, endlessly. She had been in the home, whistling the same four notes over and over, all day, every day, and almost all night every night, for the past four-and-a-half-years.

My admiration for the staff here, and their endless patience, knew no bounds.

'Fuck off with that whistling!' shouted the first lady, as everyone rolled their eyes again.

'Never mind her whistling,' whispered Joyce. 'She's a bit gone in the head, she is. You have to make allowances.'

'We will,' assured Heather.

'Because she's a bit gone in the head,' went on Joyce, revolving her finger again.

'Let's go to your room, mum,' I suggested, as I knew we were never going to have any time with her while she was seated with the others.

Mum stood up, waved goodbye to her friends, and walked towards the door with us.

'Fuck off, the lot of you!' shouted the first lady as we went.

Joyce was waving her finger around her ear again and mouthing *'She's a bit gone in the head,'* to me when I looked back.

'You mustn't pay any attention to that lot,' said mum, as we invaded the peace and quiet of the corridor.

'That's all right,' I said.

'Joyce said to me that some of them are a bit mad in here,' whispered mum, 'but don't tell anyone else I said so.'

'No we won't,' Heather agreed.

'I like to talk to Joyce,' said mum. '*She* knows what's going on.'

As we walked down the corridor, suddenly from nowhere a little old man wearing baggy trousers, a string vest and a red bandana over his head joined us. He held mum's hand without saying a word, and mum didn't say anything either; nor did they look at each other or acknowledge each other's presence in any way, they just held hands as we walked along.

When we got to mum's room we opened the door, and mum and this man went in. Mum waited by the door as the man walked over to the bed, stooped very slowly down and looked carefully under the bed.

'He's gone,' announced the little man, slowly standing up.

Mum nodded and went and sat on the bed.

'What was all that about?' I asked. 'And who is this?'

The little man in the bandana was now sitting on the side of the bed with mum.

'I want you to write a letter for me,' said mum, ignoring the question.

Mum and the little man nodded their heads together vigorously.

'There's some paper and a pen in the drawer over there,' she said, pointing to one of her bedside tables.

I knew I wouldn't be able to get any focus out of her until I did what she wanted, so I got the paper and pen.

'Someone keeps hiding under my bed,' began mum, 'and when I'm asleep, he sneaks out and steals my chocolates.'

The little man in the bandana was nodding his head furiously.

'How do you know this?' I asked.

'I can hear the sweet papers rustling in the night,' whispered mum, 'and when I do, I pull the covers up tight under my chin and pretend I'm asleep.'

I sighed.

Dear Sir,

I am writing to protest in the strongest possible terms about the man who hides under Mrs Slevin's bed at night, and comes out when she is asleep to steal her chocolates. This is a very unsatisfactory state of affairs, and is causing deep distress to Mrs Slevin, who values her chocolates above all other possessions.

I think it would be a very good idea if you informed the Sweetie Police about this matter, so that steps can be taken to apprehend the villain without further delay.

Yours faithfully,
Martin Slevin.

Mum and the little man nodded their heads together as I read the letter out. The little man wiped away a tear from his eye.

'Wonderful,' he said. It was the first word he had spoken to us.

'Now don't be getting yourself all upset, Frank,' said mum. 'Richard has written a letter now, and it will be dealt with, don't you worry.'

'This is Frank?' asked Heather, grinning.

Mum nodded, and Frank smiled.

'Frank's a fighter pilot,' announced mum proudly. 'We're getting married.'

The door opened and Joyce came in. She walked up to me and whispered, 'Don't take any notice of that lot, Richard.'

'Because they're all a bit gone in the head?' I said.

'You've noticed it too?' whispered Joyce. She rolled her finger around her ear. 'They're all a bit gone in the head.'

'Come on, Freda,' called a nurse who had followed the lady into mum's room. 'Come on out of there and let Rose have a visit in peace.'

Joyce, a.k.a. Freda, left the room quietly.

'And you, Cecil,' called the nurse.

Quick as a flash, the fighter pilot took off and was gone, shooting out of the room as though someone had shouted, 'Scramble!'

'Sorry about all that,' said the nurse. 'I'll leave you in peace with mum now.'

She shut the door behind her.

'We've brought you some chocolates,' announced Heather, handing mum the box.

'Did you manage to get them back?' asked mum.

We must have looked puzzled.

'From *him*!' mum whispered, indicating the space under her bed.

'Er… No, they're new ones,' I said.

Mum nodded. 'I'll hide them when you've gone.'

'Is everything else okay?' I asked. 'I mean, apart from the man under the bed.'

'People are very kind here,' said mum. 'I really do appreciate it.'

The door opened again and the whistling woman came in and just stood there whistling. (I call her 'the whistling woman' as I never did discover her real name, or anything else about her at all.)

'Hello,' I said.

The lady stood in the doorway with her hands on her hips. She looked directly at us, and continued to whistle her four note tune, over and over again.

A sleeve appeared in the doorway belonging to a nurse's pale blue uniform. The hand at the end of the sleeve grabbed the whistling woman's cardigan and gently pulled her backwards out of the room; as she disappeared, the whistling carried on uninterrupted.

'She's very nice,' said mum, when the whistling woman had gone. 'She used to be a professional singer.'

I never discovered if that was true or not; it didn't matter much to me, anyway.

'The grounds are beautiful here,' observed Heather, looking out of the window and changing the subject.

'I often go out there,' said mum. 'The gardener fancies me.'

She seemed to blush ever so slightly as she spoke, like a young schoolgirl.

'Does he now?' said Heather.

'But he's very respectful,' continued mum. 'He always says, "Good morning, Mrs Slevin, and how are you today?" and "You're looking very nice today, Mrs Slevin", and things like that.'

'Maybe Old Frank has a rival, then mum,' I ventured.

'He'll have to keep on his toes, won't he?' said mum, and we all laughed.

'I like Frank's bandana,' I said. 'Very trendy.'

Mum beckoned me to lean forwards, this was her signal that something very important and confidential was going to pass between us. I leaned forwards.

'He's just had his brain taken out and cleaned,' whispered mum. 'He has to wear that scarf thing until the scar on his head goes away.'

'Oh, I see,' I whispered. 'Why did he have to have his brain cleaned?'

Mum shrugged her shoulders. 'How should I know? Maybe it was dirty.'

The simple, straightforward and yet slightly faulty logic of Alzheimer's.

The door opened yet again, but this time a very smart, middle-aged lady in a dark business suit and small gold-rimmed spectacles came into the room.

'Hello,' she said brightly, striding across the room with her right hand outstretched for someone to shake. 'I'm Mrs Porter, and I'm the manager here. I'm very sorry I haven't made myself known to you before now. I was away… Bit of a family crisis.'

We all nodded that we understood, and shook hands with her in turn.

'We're very pleased with Rose, here at Charnwood House, aren't we?' said Mrs Porter looking directly at mum, who beamed a great big smile. It was like she had just been praised by the Head Teacher in front of the whole school. 'There are some papers I need you to sign, Mr Slevin. Could you drop by my office when you have finished?'

'Certainly,' I said.

When the manager left, Heather and I showed mum some of the ornaments we had brought from home to make her room more personalised. We brought some pictures of her grand-children, Rebecca and Daniel, and a few little knick-knacks that had sentimental value to mum in the past. She didn't recognise any of them, and thought the ornaments were all new.

Soon we said our goodbyes, and dropped in to see Mrs Porter on our way out.

'I just wanted to let you know that there's no money left in mum's account,' she said. 'And the hairdresser is due to arrive next Wednesday. Mum does like to have her hair done, doesn't she?'

'She does,' I said. I agreed that mum did like to have her hair done and handed over £50.

'That should keep her going for a bit,' I said.

Mrs Porter handed me a receipt.

'My mother's a lot happier here than she was at her previous home,' I said. 'We're very pleased she's been able to come here.'

'Where was she before?' asked Mrs Porter.

I mentioned the name, and her face crinkled up like a freeze-dried prune.

'Professionally, I can't really comment,' she said. 'But I guarantee you we have… ' She was searching for the right word. 'Er… Shall we say, we have *standards* here. And we are proud of our standards.'

'I agree,' I said. 'It's just a pity that all homes are not run in the same way.'

'They're supposed to be,' she said. 'But in the real world, what is supposed to happen and what really does happen are not always the same thing.'

We agreed that they were not indeed. We shook her hand again, and left. I felt that she was the sort of person you could trust your life-savings to – or, more importantly, the welfare of your mother.

The next day at work I went to the Post Office in my lunch break.

Dear Mrs Slevin,

We were shocked and dismayed to discover that your chocolates have been stolen by a person or persons unknown, who have been secreting themselves under your bed at night. Please rest assured we are doing everything in our power to bring the culprits to justice; in the meantime, please accept this box of chocolates as a small token of our esteem, and say hello to Wing Commander Frank for us.

Chief Inspector Nitram Nivels,

Coventry Sweetie Police.

21. A Secret Revealed

AS MUM'S DAYS at Charnwood House slowly turned into weeks, and then into months, she came to consider her time there in terms of her own lifespan; that is to say, she completely lost all recollection of ever having lived anywhere else.

All the years before her arrival at Charnwood ceased to mean anything to her. All the events of those years – the people who inhabited those important former times, all her family and friends, the places and happenings – all dropped their mental connections with her, one by one, until the microcosm that was Charnwood House was all she came to know and understand in the world.

The rug of her memories, as the first consultant had told me it would be almost five years before, had now been rolled up so far that only a distorted version of her childhood remained, and that childhood had all been spent in Charnwood House. It was as if she had been born there, had gone to school there, had married my dad and given birth to me there, had spent her life and career there, and now in her old age, was resigned to staying there forever, never having been anywhere else at all. Mum became fearful of the outside world, and any suggestion of her ever having to leave Charnwood House would send her into a tearful and nervous panic.

The Irish band and her shaven pal Bruno were never mentioned again; the events of the Christmas she had enjoyed so much with me were erased completely, and my own identity and history with my parents at home had dissolved utterly into the fog of her Alzheimer's. Even my father, whom mum had been married to for 60 happy years, was only a distant shadow without substance, or form. Dad had become an indistinct idea rather than a real person to her, as though she had met him in a dream the night before and now, upon waking, she could focus on his form and features no longer.

But in the midst of all this waste, this terrible loss of all things ancient, sacred and treasured, the little girl in the radiator remained as firmly rooted into mum's everyday consciousness and reality as anything could be said to be.

She spoke to the little girl every day, and when Heather and I paid our weekly visit to Charnwood House, I would watch her secretly looking towards any radiator in the building and smiling or shaking her head; clearly, the little girl inhabited not one but every radiator. Mum's lips would move very slowly and softly when she spoke to the little girl, as though they were always passing secrets between themselves, and the understanding they shared together was strictly for the two of them alone. It would be no exaggeration to state that the little girl in the radiator had become my mum's only reliable constant, a dependable anchor and friend in a vast, uncharted ocean of uncertainty, confusion and change.

One day in the late summer of 2006, Heather had asked me to drop into Charnwood House on my way home from work to deliver some toiletries, chocolates and clothes to mum.

'Give her my love,' Heather had said as I left for work that morning.

I arrived at Charnwood at around 5pm that evening, just as all the residents were having supper. I didn't like to disturb mum by arriving at meal times, and so I decided to go straight to her room and put the toiletries away for her. As I walked down the corridor from the main entrance, the whistling woman was walking up the other way towards me. At first I didn't notice anything to be different, but then I suddenly realised there was silence in the corridor. The whistling woman had stopped whistling, and was walking perfectly normally down the corridor.

'Hello,' she said as she passed me. She could have been a visitor.

I stopped dead in my tracks and looked after her. She went down the corridor and turned into the communal lounge, where my mum was having supper. A nurse saw my puzzlement. 'She stopped whistling yesterday,' she said, 'and she hasn't whistled since.'

The whistling woman never whistled again, as far as I know: for some reason, she just stopped, and that was that. One day, perhaps, we will understand the secret mechanics of dementia, and Alzheimer's in particular; but until then, there will remain a tantalising mystery, and a sad, magical enchantment entwined around the condition that fascinates all who come into contact with it like no other human ailment can.

When I entered mum's room I was shocked to see that all the little ornaments we had brought here from mum's home were damaged in some way. The little figures mum had cherished for years when I was growing up had all had their heads broken off. The porcelain flower bowl was broken into two halves, and some of her photo frames containing pictures of her grandchildren were snapped or bent. The room looked like it had been burgled by some heartless criminal, but of course that wasn't the case.

'Peggy did it,' said mum, when I questioned her later. 'Isn't she a bitch for doing that?'

I wanted to put the broken pieces into the wastepaper basket, but mum stopped me.

'It's all right,' she said. 'Frank can glue all those back together.'

'Why would Aunt Peggy do such a thing?' I asked.

Mum shrugged her shoulders. 'Who knows?' she whispered. 'Maybe she's jealous of me and Frank.'

'I've put some more clothes in your wardrobe,' I said, 'and some toiletries into the bathroom. There's some chocolates in the drawer.'

Mum stood up and went to the drawer, she took out the chocolates.

'Let's have some sweets before *he* gets hold of them!' announced mum, her eyes darting to the space under her bed.

'Is he still under there?' I asked.

'He comes and goes,' said mum. 'They can't catch him.'

I happened to have a small tube of glue in the car, which was still in there after I had fixed something the week before.

'I can glue those ornaments for you,' I said. 'Wait here and have some chocolates, mum. I'll be back in a minute.'

It was no more than a two minute walk to the car and back. When I returned to mum's room I could hear whispered voices. The bedroom door was ajar, and I peered through the gap between the door and the frame. Mum was kneeling in front of the radiator, the box of chocolates was on the floor in front of her, and she was holding out a chocolate to the radiator. I understood immediately what she was doing; she was offering a chocolate to the little girl.

I stepped into the room as softly as I could, and stood waiting quietly behind her; she had no idea I was there. Mum would take a chocolate from the box, offer it to the little girl, and then seem to freeze, her arm outstretched. After a few seconds of this, where mum would whisper something to the little girl that I couldn't hear, she would pop the chocolate into her own mouth. Then she would take another from the box, and the whole thing would start over.

Eventually, I had to speak. 'Is she still in there, mum?' I said.

'She's always going to be in there,' replied mum, over her shoulder. 'She can't get out.'

'Why can't she?' I asked, kneeling down beside her. I had become as much involved with the little girl as mum.

'It's very dark in there,' whispered mum, 'and she can't see her way out. She can't find the door, the poor little thing.'

'Is she very unhappy?' I asked. I wondered if the little girl in the radiator could be helped to escape, and whether that might have a beneficial effect on mum's Alzheimer's. It sounded completely crazy, but she believed in the little girl so much that if something good were to happen to her perhaps it might also produce benefits for my mum, too. Stranger things have happened to Alzheimer's patients than that.

'She's not very unhappy,' said mum softly. 'She's just lost in the dark, and she's confused. Sometimes she gets very frightened in there.'

'Is that why you always talk to her?' I asked quietly.

'I don't want her to be in the dark on her own,' replied mum. 'She's so little, really.'

'You've become a very good friend to her,' I said.

Mum smiled. 'She needs a good friend.'

'Do you think she's ever going to come out?' I whispered.

Mum looked at me, sadly. 'I don't see how she can,' she confessed.

She had always been very reluctant to discuss her relationship with the little girl in the radiator, and it had taken the best part of three years for her to open up this much with me about it. But this evening she seemed more willing than usual to talk about her little friend, and I decided to push the matter as far as she would be willing to allow it.

'What's she like, the little girl?' I asked.

Mum seemed to think about the question for a moment.

'She's a nice little girl,' said mum, very softly; so softly, in fact, that I could barely hear the words as they escaped her lips.

'Where does she come from, do you know?' I asked.

There was so long a pause here that I thought mum hadn't heard the question. I was about to ask it again when mum spoke. 'I know everything about her now,' she said. 'She comes from Dublin, but she can't ever go home, not now.'

'Perhaps together we could help her to escape?' I said.

'She would like that,' replied mum, 'but it's so dark in there that she could never find her way home again.'

'Has she told you that?' I asked.

Mum nodded. 'She tells me everything.'

'What does she tell you?'

I was trying to keep mum talking, to keep her attention on the little girl in the radiator, so that we could perhaps get to the bottom of this enduring mystery at last.

'She tells me lots of things,' replied mum. 'She tells me how kind to me you are, and how good to me you have been. She tells me secrets about Peggy, and about me mammy. She knows all about me, and I know all about her.'

'You've become very close then, you and this little girl,' I said.

'We're the same,' replied mum, simply.

I felt a lump swell in my throat as the penny began to drop.

'Do you know her name?' I asked. But I already knew the answer.

'Her name is Rose,' replied mum, with a sigh.

We knelt there on the floor of her room together facing the radiator in silence. As the last piece of the jigsaw puzzle suddenly snapped into place, I thought that Alzheimer's disease was the cruellest of all human ills. For it not only robs the sufferer of hope and a future, but as it goes it steals their very identity as well.

'Her name is Rose?' I said. The words caught in my throat.

Mum nodded, and continued to look at the floor.

'She's you, isn't she?' I whispered, and my eyes filled with tears that I could not hold back. 'You're the little girl in the radiator, aren't you?'

'She's trapped in the dark,' replied mum.

I thought my heart would break.

'She can't get out,' whispered mum. 'She gets so lost and confused. I've tried to help her, but I don't know how.'

I put my arm around her and she put her head against my shoulder, and we both started to sob. We stayed there on the floor of her room for a long time like that; not speaking a word, just holding each other. With the discovery at last of the identity of the little girl in the radiator had come a crashing clarity of understanding for me. I now knew why this delusion above all others had persisted through the years, and why the image of a small child, alone, frightened and abandoned in the dark, was the perfect description of the effects of Alzheimer's itself. When I finally understood that the little girl Rose in the radiator and the elderly woman Rose in the world were one and the same, I understood more about her condition than all the doctors and consultants had been able to explain in the five years since her diagnosis.

To the outside world, such fantasies are the direct result of madness and nothing the patient says or suggests can have any value. This is a great mistake. Such fantasies are rooted in the depths of the past, nearly always based on real incidents. What they say in the midst of such fantasies are not really 'delusions' at all, they are merely the retelling of real events which are now misplaced in time. I don't mean, of course, that there was ever really a little girl in a radiator; but once I understood mum's viewpoint the story made sense.

We knelt, hugged, rocked and wept together, there on the floor of her room, until we could hug and weep no more. Mum went to her bed after that, and I drove home to Heather, with my soul in shreds.

Something happened to both my mother and me that day, and even now I cannot quite understand what it was.

For mum, I think the revealing of the identity of the little girl in the radiator was almost like a sacred confession: the disclosing of a long and faithfully-held secret which unburdened her when the weight of it was finally set down.

For me, a feeling of utter foolishness engulfed me like a blanket. How could I have been so stupid? How could I have failed to guess that the little girl in the radiator and my mother were one and the same? How could I have not seen that the little girl was a pictorial representation in mum's mind of her own vulnerability, due to the wasting disease that poisoned her brain? That mum's own sense of hopelessness regarding her condition was indeed like being lost in the dark, and the radiator was merely a convenient place for the two ideas to be housed together?

The more I thought about this, the more it all made perfect sense from mum's point of view. Even though the disease was eating away her ability to function in the outside world, there was still a small part of her that was able to make sense of the condition, and represent it with a pictorial analogy to the rest of us; the fact that the rest of us were too dumb to understand it was not her fault.

A deep understanding had been forged between my mum and me with the disclosure of the identity of the little girl. I had been let into the secret, as it were, and there was a bond between us that had never been there in former years for either of us. I felt that at last there was the possibility of making some progress with mum, now that an obstacle which had stood between her and the outside world had been removed. I felt that I might be able to reach her now at some deeper level, and that the future for our relationship held a glimmer of hope.

Ironically, it was only a few weeks later that our world exploded without warning into a shower of sparks, when I received a telephone call at work from Charnwood House.

22. The Stroke

THE NURSE AT CHARNWOOD said mum had undergone 'a funny turn' and had been taken by ambulance that afternoon to the hospital at Walsgrave.

I left work early and drove straight there, trying to figure out what a 'funny turn' really meant. Had mum just experienced a slight giddiness and possibly fallen over, or was she at death's door? I arrived at reception, slightly breathless.

'Mrs Rose Slevin, admitted by ambulance this afternoon from Charnwood House nursing home?' I said to the receptionist. 'I'm her son.'

'I'll check,' she said, without looking up at me.

Behind me, a queue of people was starting to form. Most of them seemed to be lost.

'Ward 52, second floor, lifts to the right,' said the receptionist, again without bothering to look at me.

The old Walsgrave hospital had been a familiar place, where the wards had names; the replacement, built on the same site, is a massive and impersonal thing, like a small, self-contained town, and its numbered wards are only one sign of this.

I joined a queue for the two lifts. Patients, doctors and relatives crammed in together as we rose to the second floor, and I squeezed out when the doors opened. I found Ward 52 and hurried to its main reception desk.

'I'm looking for Mrs Slevin, please,' I said. 'She was admitted today. I'm her son.'

'I'll check.'

The nurse scanned a computer screen. 'Oh yes, stroke victim. Room 17. Through the double doors, turn left.'

Stroke victim.

It was the first time anyone had mentioned the word 'stroke' to me. So that was what they meant by 'a funny turn'.

I followed her instructions to Room 17, and went in.

Mum was sitting up on a narrow bed-like trolley. She looked wild-eyed and frightened. The moment she saw me she began to chatter, but the sounds she made were completely unintelligible. She looked from side to side and then back to me, her eyes darting around the room. The left side of her mouth failed to move at all when she spoke.

'Oh God,' I said. 'How are you, mum?'

I kissed her. The whole time she made frantic, panicked sounds, as though she were desperately trying to tell me something, but was unable to get the message across. I stood by the side of her bed and listened, not knowing what to do, or say.

The door opened and a nurse came in. 'Hello,' she said cheerily, 'are you a relative?'

'Yes, I'm her son,' I replied.

'I'm just going to take her blood pressure. The doctor will be along to see you in a little while.'

'Has she had a stroke?' I asked, already knowing the answer.

'The doctor will explain everything to you,' replied the nurse.

As the woman checked her blood pressure, mum continued to chatter in a language all of her own. The nurse ignored her.

'That's fine,' announced the nurse, unwrapping the Velcro band from mum's arm with a loud ripping sound. 'The doctor will be along shortly.'

I rang Heather and told her the news.

'Do you want me to come over?' she asked.

'No, there's no point,' I said. 'I'll let you know if there are any developments.'

The doctor arrived and I rang off.

'Hello,' said the doctor. 'Are you a relative?'

She looked like a 15-year-old schoolgirl – one who hadn't been to bed in a week. She brushed her hair casually back from her face as we shook hands.

'I'm her son.'

'Splendid.'

I wondered why that was splendid.

'I need to ask you some questions,' she said.

'Okay,' I replied.

She asked me the sort of things she would have normally asked mum, if mum had been able to understand the questions and the doctor had been able to understand the answers – full name, date of birth, home address, any medication, history of strokes in the family, special allergies or dietary requirements, current medical condition, and so on. I answered everything as best as I could.

'Has my mother had a stroke?' I said, finally.

'Oh yes, most definitely,' came the emphatic reply.

'What has actually happened?'

'A stroke is an episode where the blood supply to the brain has been interrupted,' she said. 'It can happen for a number of reasons and it's fairly common among people of your mother's age.'

'Is the damage permanent?'

'Too early to tell,' she replied, brushing her hair away from her face again. 'Every stroke victim deals with their condition differently. Some people recover almost immediately, some take a long time, others never recover. Some people recover partially, others make a full recovery. It all depends.'

I looked at mum, she was still chattering.

'She also has Alzheimer's,' I said.

'I thought as much,' replied the doctor. 'Your mum's admittance notes haven't arrived on the ward yet, but I thought there was dementia there.'

'What's the outlook?'

'As I say, it's too early to tell. The first 48 hours are critical. If there is going to be any major recovery then it should start to happen within the first two days. She'll be well looked after here, don't worry. We'll watch her closely.'

'I see.'

The doctor looked intently at mum. 'She's very distressed at the moment, we can give her something for that,' she said.

Then she smiled, shook my hand again, and left. I hoped she was going home to bed, but I doubted it. Within a few minutes the first nurse returned.

'I just have to give your mum something to make her feel a little easier and a bit more comfortable,' she announced brightly.

She gave my mum an injection, and mum was unconscious before the needle was removed. It was as though she had been shot.

'There, that's better, she'll sleep now,' said the nurse, and then she, too, was gone.

I stared at mum. Only a few days previously, I had felt that she and I were making progress with her dementia, after her confession as to the real identity of the little girl in the radiator. Now our little sandcastle had been hit by a tidal wave; all trace of improvement had been washed clean away, and nothing remained to suggest there had once been a sandcastle there at all.

I waited in that little room for what seemed like an eternity, although in reality it was probably an hour at the most. Mum never stirred and no-one came back. In the end I returned to the front desk.

'Can you tell me what's happening with Mrs Slevin in Room 17, please?' I asked.

The nurse looked at her computer screen. 'I'll check for you,' she said.

She scanned her system looking for the data that referred to 'unit Slevin'. It wasn't there.

'What's happening with Mrs Stevens?' she called to a colleague nearby.

'Slevin, not Stevens,' I said.

More checking.

Then, from the colleague, 'She's waiting for a bed on the ward. She'll be assessed and the consultant will review her in the morning. Give us a ring after 10 o'clock and we should know more by then.'

The new 'program unit Mrs Slevin' hadn't been uploaded yet, so the set of statistics that was my mother was just left unconscious on a trolley-bed until the great programmer was ready to enter her into the system. Maybe at the end of the day we're all just numbers on someone's spreadsheet.

I went home to Heather.

I took the next day off work, and we both waited at home until after 10 o'clock as I had been instructed. Then I rang the hospital.

The number rang… and rang… and rang… and rang…

'What's happening?' asked Heather, after five minutes.

'Nothing's happening,' I replied. 'It's just ringing and ringing. No-one's answering.'

She went to make us a cup of coffee and when she returned a few minutes later I was still listening to the ringing tone. By now, I'd been hanging on for almost 10 minutes.

'This is ridiculous,' said Heather. 'What if it was urgent?'

'It *is* urgent!' I replied.

'But what if it was an emergency?' she asked.

'I suppose I'd have to ring 999,' I replied.

It's beyond frustrating to sit there with a telephone pressed to your ear listening to a mechanical tone repeat itself time after time with nothing else happening. You are tempted to replace the receiver and dial again; the problem is, if you're in a queue you lose your slot and rejoin the queue at the far end. Of course, if you're not told you're in a queuing system in the first place then you don't know what to do, so you continue to sit there until either someone answers the phone, you get cut off, you die, or the world comes to an end.

'I'll make some toast,' said Heather.

When she came back with a plate of toast for me the telephone at Walsgrave hospital main switchboard had still not been answered. I had now been waiting for 22 minutes.

'Put the phone down,' said Heather, 'and we'll drive over now.'

Suddenly, a voice came through the receiver, so harsh and unexpected that it startled me.

'Walsgrave Hospital.'

'I've been waiting for someone to answer the telephone for nearly half an hour,' I said. 'I thought you had all died up there!'

'There's no need for that attitude. We *are* busy here, you know. It's a hospital.'

'I know it's a hospital,' I replied, 'I just thought you might be able to be a bit more efficient on the switchboard, that's all.'

The line just went dead, suddenly replaced with the dialling tone. The receptionist had cut me off.

I stared into the plastic receiver, as though by giving the telephone a really hateful look I might actually scare the thing into being more co-operative next time.

'She's put the phone down!' I gasped, incredulously.

'What did you have a go at her for?' said Heather.

I put the receiver back on the cradle.

'Come on,' announced Heather, putting her coat on. 'Let's go over there.'

We entered the hospital grounds and followed the snaking lane around the perimeter until we eventually came to the car parks, where we drove around in circles several times until we finally found a space; it was almost full, and it was only 11am. We walked to the main entrance. Outside the revolving doors, a number of people were standing smoking in the rain. I noticed one man dressed in pale blue pyjamas and red slippers, a cigarette in one hand and a steel upright stand supporting a saline drip in the other. His pyjamas were wet through. There was also a very elderly woman sitting in a wheelchair in her dressing gown and slippers who looked like she had been smoking out there all morning. Over our heads, a recorded metallic voice boomed: 'Walsgrave Hospital is now a non-smoking hospital. This includes the grounds and car parks. The hospital administrators would like to thank everyone for their continued co-operation with this policy.'

We walked through the large revolving doors and went around to the right of the reception desk towards the elevators. As we passed by, a telephone was ringing but no-one was answering it: a gaggle of women sat at the desk gossiping and joking, ignoring the insistent sound.

I started to walk towards the desk. I meant to ask the people who were paid to answer the telephone if they understood how important the call they were ignoring might be to someone, but Heather read my mind.

'Leave it, Martin,' she said, 'it doesn't matter.'

193

'It does matter, though,' I said, but I walked past.

There was a huge queue for the lifts – patients in wheelchairs, a man on a trolley with a tube up his nose, and several visitors holding bunches of flowers. When the doors opened, there was a rush as we all piled in. I smelled lilies.

'Doors closing,' intoned a metallic voice, as the doors shut.

'First floor,' announced the voice, as the doors opened again. 'Doors opening.'

Helpful, I thought.

'Going down?' asked the man at the front of the crowd on the first floor.

'No, going up!' shouted someone at the back of the lift.

'Doors closing,' announced the robotic voice.

The lift jerked upwards.

'I wanted that floor!' said an elderly man with a walking stick, who was standing behind me. 'It didn't give me enough time!'

A few people shook their heads and tutted. The old man managed to push his way nearer to the front of the crowd.

'Second floor,' said the voice. 'Doors opening.'

The doors opened. A crowd at the second floor pressed forwards and blocked the exit of those already in the lift, including us. There was a lot of polite pushing and shoving. The old man behind me still didn't manage to get out.

'Doors closing.'

'Oh, bugger!' he shouted, as the doors closed in front of him again.

Heather and I left the elevator, and began to walk down the endless corridor to Ward 52.

We entered the ward and went up to the reception desk.

'We've come to see Mrs Slevin,' I said to the nurse on reception.

'I'm sorry, but it's not visiting time yet,' she smiled.

'I tried calling first,' I replied, 'but after waiting half-an-hour for someone to answer the telephone we gave up and came down in person.'

I didn't tell her the receptionist had hung up on me.

'Sorry about that,' apologised the nurse. I suppose it wasn't her fault.

'So how is my mum?' I asked.

'You've missed the consultant,' she said. 'His round was at 10 o'clock.'

'Yes, I know,' I said. 'I was asked to call after then so that I could get more information.'

'Oh, I see,' she replied, and started to look around for someone else to talk to.

A man in a white coat and a stethoscope around his neck came up to us.

'Can I help you?' he asked. He was smiling broadly at us, too; it was almost as though they'd all been on a course.

'I just want to know how my mother is. Mrs Rose Slevin, admitted from Charnwood nursing home yesterday. She had a stroke.'

'Ah, yes,' he said. 'She's very comfortable just now.'

'But I want to talk to someone about what's happened to her,' I said. 'Are you a doctor?'

'Yes, I am,' he replied, still smiling.

'So... What's happened to her?' I asked.

'I don't really know,' he beamed. 'She's not one of my patients. Let me have a look at the notes.'

'Whose patient is she?' asked Heather.

'She's under Mr... Mmmmmm... Not really sure,' he said. He was still smiling, though a little less broadly now. 'I'll find out for you.'

The doctor leafed through mum's notes. 'She hasn't had a stroke,' he said.

'She hasn't?' Heather and I looked at each other.

'She's been down for a scan, and there was no sign of a stroke whatsoever,'

Now he looked more radiant than ever.

'So what has happened?' I asked.

'If you ring this number you can speak to the consultant's secretary who is in charge of your mother's case,' he said, grinning from ear to ear.

I wondered why the consultant's secretary was in charge of my mother.

He was scribbling down a telephone number on a small notepad he took from his coat pocket.

'You can make an appointment to see the consultant who can tell you everything you need to know,' he said. He looked so pleased with himself it was as though he had just discovered the cure for the common cold.

'Can't you just tell me?' I asked.

'She's not my patient,' he repeated, and again the beatific smile seemed to fade just a little.

'Where is she now?' asked Heather.

'Ah,' he said brightly. 'She's just around the corner in room four.' He could answer that one.

The result of speaking to several nurses and a doctor, then, was that we knew little more about what had actually happened to mum than we had before we had arrived.

We wandered off to find room four.

23. Nil By Mouth

WE ENTERED THE ROOM and stood there in silence.

Mum was asleep, but sitting almost upright on a bed. She was wearing one of those hospital gowns which ties at the neck and sides and is open all the way down the back; it was in red and yellow and had the words: *Walsgrave Hospital do not remove* repeated over and over across it, as though previous patients had taken theirs home, perhaps to wear out to a nice restaurant.

She looked 10 years older than she had the day before. Her mouth hung down on the left hand side, and I knew she was in serious trouble. How did I know this? Her hair was a mess. In 50 years I had never seen her with her hair not looking immaculate. Even as her condition deteriorated at Charnwood House, this had held true. She believed a man under her bed was eating her chocolates at night, she thought she was pregnant and going to marry a fighter pilot, and she thought that I was her brother and worked as a council bullfighter; but she never missed getting her hair done every Wednesday.

A plastic tube ran from a needle inserted into the back of her left hand up to a saline drip over her head. Above her bed a white plastic sign, hung on a nail, simply stated: NIL BY MOUTH.

Beneath the white blanket which covered her, her legs were exposed below the knee, and I winced when I saw how slender and stick-like they were. She had never been a big woman, but now she was a waif: frail and elderly, alone and very vulnerable.

Mum opened her eyes, looked at me and smiled.

'Hi mum,' I said, as I leaned forwards and kissed her on the forehead. 'How are you doing?'

Bloody stupid question really.

She smiled at me and nodded.

A different doctor came into the room.

'I just want to do a few simple tests,' he explained.

He gripped mum's right hand in his and asked her to squeeze his hand as hard as she could. I could see her fingers tighten around his palm.

'That's very good, Mrs Slevin,' he said, gently replacing her hand on the blanket by her side. 'Now the other hand.'

He put mum's left hand in his, and again asked her to squeeze his palm as hard as she could. There was no perceptible movement in her fingers.

'As hard as you can, Mrs Slevin,' he repeated.

Still her fingers did not move. Even from where I was standing at the other side of the bed, I could tell there was no pressure there.

He put her hand back, moved to the end of the bed, straightened mum's feet and put the palm of his hand against the sole of her right foot.

'Push hard, Mrs Slevin, please,' he said, and I could see mum's toes curl, as she straightened her leg, and pushed his hand away.

'Very good, indeed,' he said, 'and now the other foot. Push against me as hard as you can, if you please, Mrs Slevin.'

There was almost no movement at all. No toe curling and no pressure.

'Try again, Mrs Slevin,' he said, 'push hard.'

Nothing.

He moved to the top of the bed and produced a small torch from his top pocket. He shone it twice into both of mum's eyes.

'Mmm,' he said to himself.

It's funny how the sound 'Mmm' can convey so much concern. It really doesn't mean anything, it isn't even a proper word, but when I heard it, my heart sank.

'Now I want you to smile a great big smile for me, Mrs Slevin,' he said. 'Give me the biggest grin you can. Come on now, you can do it!'

Mum smiled on the right side of her mouth only. The left side stayed put.

'Mmm,' he said again, and started to make some notes.

'What's the story?' I asked.

Without replying he walked slowly out into the ward, and we followed him. He closed the door, so that we were all outside mum's room. There was a telephone ringing and ringing somewhere on the ward; no-one was moving towards it. I thought about the relative on the other end.

'Who are you?' he asked.

'I'm her son,' I said.

'Well, your mother has suffered a very severe stroke,' he said. 'It has killed the swallowing reflex in her throat, and has paralysed the left side of her body, head arm, side and leg. I'm afraid it is very serious.'

'We've just been told that she hasn't had a stroke,' I said, clutching at the proverbial straw.

'The scan didn't show anything,' said Heather.

'Sometimes that's the case,' he explained. 'Sometimes, if the scan is done straight away after the stroke, nothing shows up. Sometimes it takes a few days for the bruising on the brain to appear. I am confident that, if we repeated the scan in the next few days, the stroke would be there.'

'I see,' I nodded.

'A stroke is an attack on the brain,' he went on. 'Because the brain controls everything we do, and all of our senses, wherever the stroke hits the brain it impairs those functions which are controlled by that particular area of the brain.'

I nodded slowly.

'In your mother's case, the stroke occurred in an area of the brain that controls left side body movement, and the swallowing reflex; it has damaged that part of your mother's brain, and therefore those functions are currently lost to her.'

'Will she get them back?' asked Heather.

'Too early to tell,' he replied. 'Some people make a full recovery after a stroke, others make only a partial recovery in time, others make no recovery at all. The first few days are critical. If progress is going to be made, it usually starts to show within the first couple of days.'

'That's today,' I said.

'We mustn't give up hope,' he said.

As soon as he said that I felt that there was no hope.

'I'll leave you now,' he said quietly, and walked away down the ward.

We went back into the room.

Mum was asleep again.

A nurse came into the room.

'I just need to take Rose's blood pressure,' she announced.

'The doctor says she's lost the swallowing reflex,' I said. 'How will she be able to eat?'

'What a shame,' said the nurse. 'When that happens we feed them through a tube, it goes up the nose and down directly into the stomach. If it's going to be long-term, then we fit a peg.'

'What's a peg?' asked Heather.

'It's a very simple medical procedure where we insert a valve called a peg into the wall of the stomach, and attach the feeding tube that way. It's a lot more comfortable for them than having a tube continually stuck up your nose.'

'Could I take the telephone number of the ward?' I asked, thinking about waiting another half-an-hour for someone to answer the telephone at the switchboard in the morning, 'so I could come directly through to here, and avoid the main switchboard?'

'Of course you can,' she said, brightly. 'I'll write the number down for you.'

The nurse scribbled some digits on a scrap of paper and handed it to me.

Heather and I waited in room four for another hour or so; mum didn't wake, and we went home.

The next morning I rang the ward.

The phone rang and rang, and rang and rang. After 20 minutes, someone answered it.

'Walsgrave Hospital.'

I tried to remain calm and to give the receptionist no excuse to put down the telephone on me again.

'I'm ringing to see how Mrs Slevin spent the night,' I said.

'What ward is she on?'

I was confused.

'Your ward, Ward 52,' I said.

'This is the main switchboard.'

I had to stifle the rising scream inside me.

'I have been ringing the ward number directly,' I replied, as patiently and politely as I could.

'If the ward doesn't answer within so many rings the call automatically diverts back to the switchboard.'

'Can you please put me through to Ward 52?' I asked very softly.

'Hold the line please.'

The telephone ringing tone started to repeat, and repeat and repeat.

'For Christ's sake!' I shouted into the receiver.

Ten minutes later, the phone was answered.

'Ward 10.'

'What?' I gasped, 'I wanted Ward 52!'

'I'll transfer you back,' said the voice.

The phone began to ring and ring again. I waited and waited, the frustration welling up inside me like a tidal wave. Fifteen minutes later, the call was finally answered. By this time I had been trying to get through to mum's ward for 45 minutes. The voice was one that I had come to hate.

'Walsgrave Hospital.'

I was back at the switchboard again.

'OH, FUCK OFF!' I shouted.

The line immediately went dead. Brrrrrrrrrrrrrrrrrrrrr. I slammed the receiver down onto the cradle.

'I'll get my coat,' sighed Heather.

I called into work and told them I wouldn't be in for a few days at least. Then we drove over to the hospital again.

In the last few years in Britain there has been an alarming and disturbing rise in the number of assaults carried out by members of the public against hospital staff. No-one could justify or condone this, but having experienced first-hand the way some hospitals are run I can understand it. When I arrived at Walsgrave that morning I was ready to kill someone.

We went back up in the elevator to Ward 52.

'I've come to see how Mrs Slevin is today,' I said through gritted teeth to the nurse at the desk.

'I'll check for you,' she replied. 'I've only just come on duty.'

She scanned her computer screen and obviously couldn't find mum.

'Where's Mrs Slevin?' she asked a colleague behind her.

The colleague shrugged her shoulders.

Heather walked down to room four, and then came back.

'Her room's empty,' said Heather.

'Where's Mrs Slevin?' asked the nurse at the desk to a passing doctor.

'She's been transferred to Ward 38,' he said, without looking over or breaking his stride.

'She's on Ward 38,' announced the nurse brightly.

We nodded and went back to the lifts.

We found mum on Ward 38, lying flat on her back, fast asleep. Her NIL BY MOUTH sign had followed her down, and was again hanging over her head. A plastic feeding tube had been inserted up her nostril, and a blue plastic mask covered her nose and mouth. I could tell they were also giving her oxygen.

'The oxygen levels in her bloodstream are a little low,' explained a nurse when I asked about it. 'So we're giving her oxygen through the mask to help her to breathe more easily.'

I noticed mum's left leg was bent at the knee, so that the sole of her foot was touching her right knee. I tried to straighten the leg but it wouldn't budge. Mum woke when I moved the leg, it was obviously painful for her to have it moved.

'That leg has become rigid since the stroke,' said a nurse. 'We've made an appointment for the physiotherapist to come and see her about it.'

It was now the third day since the stroke and I was keen to see if there had been any improvement in mum's condition.

I took her left hand in mine.

'Squeeze my hand as hard as you can, mum,' I said.

Nothing.

'Come on, you're not trying,' I said. 'Squeeze hard.'

The pressure of her fingers increased around mine; but it was so gentle that it was like the touch of a butterfly's wing.

I put her hand back onto the blanket.

'The consultant wants to have a word with you, Mr Slevin,' said a nurse as she came by. 'He'll be down in a minute.'

Heather and I looked at each other; we didn't know whether this was a good sign or a bad one. I think we both feared the worst.

The consultant came into the ward. He was a very tall, grey-haired gentleman in a dark suit and what looked like a cricket club tie in red and blue stripes knotted tightly at his neck. He was carrying a clipboard. As soon as he appeared, the nurses all seemed to look very busy. The telephone which had been incessantly ringing in the corridor was suddenly answered. When the call was finished the receiver was replaced. It rang again and was answered immediately. It was obvious that this man mattered.

'Hello,' he said, and introduced himself. 'We're going to have to fit a peg into your mother's stomach so that we can feed her more easily. The problem with feeding someone nasally is that the throat can become sore on the inside and it can lead to an infection.'

Heather and I nodded.

'But because it is an operation, even a very minor one, we do need you to authorise the procedure, as the next of kin, as it were.'

We nodded again.

'Any questions?'

I felt like asking him why nobody ever answered the telephone, but I knew that wasn't the sort of thing he had in mind.

'There doesn't seem to be much improvement since the stroke,' said Heather.

He shook his head. 'No.'

'What's the long-term prognosis?' I asked.

He took a deep breath. 'It's difficult to say with any degree of certainty. We can make your mother comfortable at least.'

'It's not good, though is it?' I asked. I wanted someone to give me a straight answer.

He shook his head again. 'No.'

We shook hands and he left.

Mum had the peg fitted the following week, and was fed through a tube for the rest of her life.

During this time there was an outbreak of MRSA at the hospital. In an effort to combat this, the hospital authorities restricted visiting time to only one hour in the evenings, from 7pm to 8pm. This caused huge traffic jams in the car park both coming in and going out, and added to the general frustration felt by most relatives when they finally managed to arrive at the hospital.

I remember on one occasion arriving at 7pm, only to have to queue up in the car park for 20 minutes so that I didn't actually arrive on the ward until nearly 7.30pm; half my time with mum was already gone. I hadn't been at her bedside for five minutes when two young trainee nurses arrived, announced they were going to give mum a bed bath, and asked me to leave the room. This had happened once before and I had reluctantly agreed. By the time they had finished, I had five minutes left of my one hour. This time I would not comply so meekly.

'Hold on a minute,' I said. 'I only get one hour a day here. Why do you have to bathe her in my one hour? Why can't you give her a bath after visiting time?'

The request seemed reasonable to me.

'We have to do things to a schedule,' one of them replied.

'Not tonight, you're not,' I said. 'You have her 23 hours a day, I have her for one. Bathe her in your time, not in mine!'

'I'll have to speak to my supervisor,' she replied.

'Speak to who you like,' I said, firmly, 'but don't come back until after I've gone at eight o'clock!'

They gave me an injured look and wheeled the trolley away. Word must have gone around about me, because they didn't come back, and no-one ever bothered me at visiting time again. Before mum became ill, if I had ever felt that my rights were being infringed in some way, I would generally say nothing: better to have a peaceful life. Now, when it's justified, I complain, all the time, about everything, to everyone, and I always win. When you're forced to fight someone else's battles for them because they are helpless, it makes you more assertive and determined to redress injustices.

Mum stayed in Walsgrave for the next 10 weeks with no visible improvement at all. Her swallowing reflex never returned, nor did the movement of the left side of her face or body. Her ability to speak was also severely impaired, to the point where it became impossible to understand a word she was saying.

Towards the end of June 2007, a member of staff from Charnwood House came out to the hospital to assess her condition. It was decided that as the stroke had left her bed-ridden, and she required full-time nursing care, Charnwood would not be able to have her back. They were sorry, but they simply didn't have the facilities to cope with someone in mum's condition.

They asked us to call in to collect mum's personal things. It was time to find somewhere else to take her.

24. Third Home

THE SOCIAL WORKER had re-established contact with us, and we told her that it would be more convenient if mum could be placed in a nursing home nearer to where we now lived. She told us that should not be a problem, and said she would come back to us with a list of suitable places for us to visit in a few days.

She came back with just one. 'There's a shortage of beds at the moment,' she told us. Once again, it was take it or leave it.

We decided to go and have a look the following weekend. It wasn't all that far away, and as we pulled up outside I was pleased with what I saw. Nice flower beds, no litter on the ground, the windows were clean and sparkling: it gave a good first impression.

'Looks nice,' observed Heather, as we made our way towards the front door.

The door was opened by the manageress; she wasn't pleased to see us. 'I've only just been told you were coming,' she said, testily. 'I should have more notice than this.'

'I'm sorry about that,' I said, although I hadn't made the appointment so I had nothing to be sorry about.

'Not your fault,' she said, softening. 'Social Services again.' She waved her arm along the corridor. 'Go through.'

We found ourselves in a gloomy corridor with a dark red, faded carpet, and cream walls on either side that could have used a fresh coat of paint. There were small plastic vases dotted here and there, sprouting equally plastic flowers with dusty petals.

'We have two rooms available,' she said. 'Follow me, and I'll show them to you.'

She marched down the corridor, swinging her arms as she went, without once looking back. I wondered if she had ever been in the army.

'This one,' she announced, standing aside and pushing the door open.

We stepped meekly into the room. It was like a prison cell. There was one table, one chair and one bed, and no other furniture at all. It was painted in 1960s surgical green, and the whole place smelled of disinfectant. Outside the ground floor window, some thoughtful architect had pencilled in the perimeter so that the only view any poor, bed-ridden patient would have for the rest of their days was of a big, red brick wall. My heart sank.

'Follow me,' she announced, and marched off again before we could even talk about it. We followed her back down the corridor.

'And this one,' she said, swinging another door open.

This was slightly better. The view from the window was of a small grassed area, with a rose bower over a small fish pond. Otherwise it was the same as the other, apart from one slight difference: there was a little old man in the bed.

'Don't mind him,' she announced loudly. 'He'll be gone tomorrow.'

For one horrible moment I thought she meant he was going to die in the morning.

The little old man looked over and smiled a toothless smile at us.

'Aren't you, Ted, going tomorrow?' she shouted.

Ted managed a wave and then fell back on the bed.

Heather and I looked at each other. I don't know which of us was the more horrified, or dumbstruck.

'Which do you prefer?' asked the manageress. 'This one's got the better view.'

'Where is Ted going?' I said. I had to ask it.

'Birmingham, nearer his relatives. Which room?'

'This one,' we said together.

'Fine, some paperwork, back to the office,' and she marched back the way we had come.

We trotted after her in line, like two little ducklings. As we all marched down the corridor I caught myself hoping Ted would make it.

We completed the paperwork and that was it, mum had a new home.

We sat in the car afterwards talking.

'Not like Charnwood, was it?' I said.

Heather shook her head. 'I always thought these places were pretty much all the same. They're not, some are really nice, and some are terrible. I had no idea it was like this.'

'Neither had I,' I confessed.

'She won't take any nonsense, anyway,' said Heather. 'I bet the staff are kept on their toes.'

'I bet,' I agreed.

How wrong we both were.

The following day we spoke to the social worker and told her we had agreed for mum to be moved there. I still wasn't sure about the place but there was nowhere else, and as mum now required full-time professional nursing care we couldn't have her back at home.

'I'll make all the arrangements,' said the social worker, and that was that.

Mum was moved by ambulance from Walsgrave Hospital on the following Wednesday, and Heather and I were going out to see her on the Sunday. We used the few days in between to gather up some more things to take with us – toiletries and new nightclothes, mainly. By this point, I was literally exhausted – after years of looking after my mother, and now this new stress and upset – and we decided to use those few days to go away. We would drive to the east coast, and visit Heather's parents; the break would do us both the world of good. I took some holiday from work, we carelessly packed a couple of bags, and drove out of the Midlands the following morning.

Getting away from mum was like a breath of fresh air. I know that sounds terribly selfish and cold, and for that I apologise, but sometimes you really need to break the bonds of responsibility, for your own wellbeing. Once refreshed, you'll have the strength to carry on again; if you never get a break, never get a reprieve from the suffering and responsibility of care, then eventually your own health will begin to suffer, and with it your ability to help your loved one.

We headed to the coast slowly, taking in the countryside as we went and planning to stop for lunch on the way. But we caught ourselves talking about mum all the way through lunch, and for most of the rest of the journey. Her Alzheimer's had occupied my thoughts every single day for the past five years, and Heather's for the past two. This was our first time away from it, and it was very difficult to let go, to talk about something else, to have a life outside the disease. At the beginning of this book, I said that Alzheimer's reaches out from the patient and grips whoever comes into contact with it, and that was certainly true of us.

We arrived in Skegness in the early evening and made ourselves comfortable at Heather's parents' house. We hadn't seen them for about six months, so we spent the rest of that evening telling them all about mum. They were fascinated with the anecdotes, as most people are, especially the elderly, and we found ourselves at midnight trying to talk about something else. A local pub shut at 1am, so we went there for the last hour. We drank in the bar and talked about mum's new home.

The next day we walked on the beach like a couple of kids. We found another bar and virtually moved in, drinking and chatting all day and most of the night; we laughed at mum's antics when she lived at home, we laughed about poor Bruno's shaved bum, and we reminisced about the nice people we had met at Charnwood House, both patients and staff. We tried to whistle the whistling woman's four-note tune, but neither of us could get it exactly right, and we tried to remember the letters I had written on mum's behalf to everyone from the leader of Coventry City Council, complaining about sharks in the swimming baths, to the manageress of Charnwood House, complaining about the way they dragged mum's room-mate out of bed every morning by her feet. We laughed and talked, and temporarily we laid the burden down. As the hours wore on, though, we became melancholic with the drink, and we cursed the fates for allowing such a nice old lady to develop so cruel and spiteful a condition. We agreed that if either of us were ever to contract the dreaded 'A' ourselves, then the other one would shoot them dead as soon as the first symptoms appeared. It's amazing what you'll agree to after you've been drinking all day long. We stumbled and danced along the beach on the way home, and it was about three o'clock in the morning when we sneaked in.

The few days we spent with Heather's parents at the coast were delightful for us. We drank too much, slept too little and laughed just the right amount. We put Walsgrave Hospital, Charnwood House and the new home behind us for a precious few days, and I think we both needed it.

On the Saturday morning we visited the local market and bought a few nice things for mum; a pink cardigan, and a silver photograph frame; I was going to put her grandchildren's pictures in it for her. We said goodbye to Heather's folks, and drove back into our reality. As we drew closer to Nuneaton, our cheerfulness evaporated. The nearer we came back to home, the more we began to resume our former roles as sober, sensible carers. Our day in the pub suddenly seemed like a lifetime ago.

We got back at around 5pm. At 7pm the telephone rang; it was the new home.

'Mrs Slevin had another stroke an hour ago, and has been rushed into George Eliot Hospital in Nuneaton. I think you should go there straight away.'

We hadn't even unpacked our bags. We walked straight out of the door again and got back into the car.

25. Second Stroke

THE GEORGE ELIOT is the main hospital in Nuneaton, and is named after the Victorian novelist who was born in the town. I liked the place because the wards have names and not numbers; I have come to feel that if they bother to name the wards, then they are more likely to see the patients as names, too – that is, as real people. If the wards merely have numbers then so do the patients, and they end up being processed like so much impersonal data.

We pulled into the car park of the Accident and Emergency section, and went in.

'Can I help you?' asked the receptionist, smiling at me.

'We've come to see Mrs Slevin, she was admitted today,' said Heather.

The lady nodded. 'The doctor will be with you in a moment. If you go through those doors to the left and take a seat in the relatives' waiting room, he won't be long.'

We followed her directions, took a seat and waited.

'This can't be good news,' I said.

'Wait until we hear what the doctor has to say,' Heather replied, sensibly.

The doctor came in. He was young and fresh-faced, he had a confident air about him, and he smiled broadly at both of us. We shook hands with him, and he closed the door, and sat down.

'Mrs Slevin's notes from Walsgrave Hospital haven't arrived here yet, so I don't know anything about this lady's medical history,' he began. 'I wanted to speak to you first. What can you tell me about her?'

We relayed mum's history as best as we could, from the time of the previous stroke at Charnwood House up until a few days ago when Heather and I had gone to the coast.

'I see,' he said when we had finished. 'Mrs Slevin has suffered a second stroke. That often happens when the first stroke has been

211

severe. We have admitted her on to Alexandra Ward, and you will be able to see her, and stay with her as often and for as long as you wish. Don't feel you have to adhere to the posted visiting times.'

'It doesn't look good then?' I asked.

'Your mother is extremely ill,' he said.

We nodded.

'What can you tell me about the nursing home she has just come from?' he asked.

'Not a lot, really,' I said. 'She only just moved in there a few days ago. She was in Walsgrave for about 10 weeks before that. Why do you ask?'

I had the strangest feeling there was something he wasn't telling me.

'She was not admitted in a favourable condition,' he replied. 'The nurse who first admitted her commented on her condition.'

'What do you mean?' asked Heather. 'What condition?'

'The admitting nurse wrote some comments in the admittance book, which is a very unusual thing for a nurse to do. I think she was covering herself.'

'I still don't understand,' I said. 'What was mum's condition when she arrived here?'

'I didn't see her personally,' he said, 'but the notes written by the admitting nurse state that she was covered in faeces. Some of it had dried onto her legs, and looked as though it had been there for some time. There was also dried faeces under her fingernails, again indicating that she had not been washed in some time. Also the feeding peg on her stomach was caked in dried blood, again indicating a lack of personal care.'

I thought I was going to be sick.

'I'm sorry to have to tell you this,' he said. 'You can go through and see her now.'

He stood up, shook hands with us again, and left us alone. We sat together in stunned silence. While Heather and I were enjoying ourselves at the seaside, mum had been neglected in the home to which we had entrusted her. They hadn't even bothered to keep her clean; even her basic personal hygiene needs had been neglected. I felt a rage begin to rise up inside me that even now I can hardly explain or contain. We went onto the ward in silence.

Mum was lying on a bed as we expected. Her skin was a pale grey colour, and her hair was a mess. All the immediate and obvious signs were bad, even to a layman like myself.

NIL BY MOUTH had followed her, and it hung again over her head in plain black text on a white card; a message of instruction, like NO SMOKING, or EXIT.

She had a tube again running from the back of her hand up to a saline drip, and another running from a liquid feed bag, to the newly cleaned, and sanitised peg in her stomach. A machine to her left monitored something critical as its little green line rose and fell with her heartbeat and breathing, and she gasped for breath once again through a blue plastic mask, which covered her nose and mouth.

I felt so sorry for her.

As we stood by her bedside, her eyes slowly opened, and she looked at me, but there were no signs of recognition there, and no smile followed the stare. I got the impression that mum knew someone was standing beside her, but she had no way of telling who that person was, or in what capacity they stood in relation to her. She simply looked at me, and then looked away.

'Hi mum,' I whispered, and kissed her gently on the forehead. 'How are you feeling?'

She turned her head to look at me again, gave me the same quizzical stare, and then returned her gaze to the ceiling.

I brushed her hair away from her face with my hand, and her forehead felt cold and clammy.

'Hello, Rose,' whispered Heather gently, bending over the bed. 'You're in hospital, in Nuneaton.'

Mum turned her eyes to look at Heather, but there was no sign of recognition in them at all. She opened her mouth to speak, and a faint, strangled gasp came out. It was barely audible, and then it faded away into silence, even though her lips continued to move for the next few seconds.

This was the last attempt at audible communication my mother ever made; the latest stroke had effectively killed her powers of speech.

I thought how sad that was. She had always loved to gossip and chat – she'd spend hours with her neighbours and friends, just passing the time in joyful conversation. Even during her time in Charnwood House, when the things she said to us made no logical sense, she was still able to enjoy the ebb and flow of the banter, and participate in the conversation. This had allowed her to remain connected to the world, even if that world was confusing and even frightening. The cruelty of Alzheimer's disease increases proportionately as its grip intensifies. As the time passes, it robs its sufferer of more and more of their natural faculties, until it renders them down to a shell, a hollow husk of wheat, with the vitality and substance that once made them whole blown away on the ever-strengthening breezes of dementia.

This was the beginning of a period that I can only now come to describe as The Long Wait.

* * * * *

We came to mum's bedside almost every evening for the next three months, and we waited. Exactly what we were waiting for is hard to define in retrospect. Maybe it was for some small sign of improvement, although I think we both knew in our hearts that the situation was hopeless. If there had been no sign of recovery after the first stroke, how could we honestly expect one after the second? Maybe we were waiting for the medical staff to give us some concrete assurance that there was either hope, or no hope at all; they could give us neither. Maybe we were waiting for mum to fail at last and to pass away. Or maybe we were just waiting for something to change; it hardly ever did.

In the first week I again took more time off work than I was really due, and slept most nights in the chair by mum's bedside. She lay there on the bed like a statue, coarsely gasping for each and every breath through her oxygen mask. I would fall asleep for a while, but any slight change in the rhythm of her breathing would immediately awaken me again and I would stare at her for a sign of life. Her breathing would then resume its staggered tempo, and I would fall asleep again, only for the whole process to repeat 20 minutes later. This cycle recurred I don't know how many times throughout each night, and, at the end of the first week, I felt that either I would have to go home to my own bed, or the nurses would end up getting me a bed in the ward as another patient. So I went home.

We came back every evening and waited. Nothing changed.

Slowly, over the course of the first month, the nurses said that mum was beginning to need the oxygen mask less and less, and eventually they removed the mask altogether and allowed her to breathe unassisted. A red mark had appeared across the bridge of her nose where the mask had rested.

Over the second month her body weight increased very slightly, and her skin lost that tragic pale grey colour, as a pink sheen returned to her face. This one single change in the colour shading of her facial skin made her look five years younger, and a whole lot healthier.

Over the course of the third month, she began to focus on the world again. She would open her eyes and look about the room. She would seem to take an interest in her surroundings, and, although she never spoke again, she did seem to appreciate what was happening around her. Mum would look about the room at the comings and goings of the staff and the visitors. She would occasionally glance at me, but there was no recognition behind the glance, it was just a glance, nothing more. She would look over to the radiator though, and smile. Only mum, Heather and I knew why, and the little girl's secret was safe with us.

Towards the end of the third month, another consultant spoke to us.

'There is very little more we can do for your mother here,' he said. 'I am sorry to put it so bluntly, but we do need the bed space now, and I think your mum would be better off in a nursing home, sooner rather than later.'

It was time for mum to move on again. She was like a geriatric gypsy.

The social worker got in touch with us again, and said that mum would need a new place to stay.

'She's not going back to that hellhole she was in before,' I said. 'They didn't even understand the first thing about personal hygiene.'

'Of course not,' she said. 'I'll find you somewhere else.'

'No, I'll do the finding,' I said. 'After our experience with the last place, I'm not going to be rushed in to sending mum anywhere I haven't checked out properly first.'

'Well, time is short, Mr Slevin,' she said, her voice had lost its self-assured quality by now.

'No, it isn't,' I said. 'I won't be pressured, either. I'm going to contact all the nursing homes in the area, and then I'll visit them one by one, and when I've made my choice, then I'll agree to have her moved, and not before. And if they don't like that here, because they have to keep her for a few weeks longer, then tough luck.'

'Oh, yes, you're right, of course,' she agreed, and that was the end of the conversation.

No matter who I upset, no matter whose schedule I disrupted, no matter whose plans I spoiled, I knew my mother wasn't going into another nursing home that I hadn't checked out thoroughly. And if that took time, then it took time; people would just have to get used to it, and make other arrangements. I knew she was well looked-after where she was, and I was in no hurry to move her again, no matter how short they were of bed space.

26. Fourth Home

I USED THE INTERNET and the local telephone directory to make a list of all the nursing homes within a 10-mile radius of where we lived.

There were 72. A lot of them had their own websites, and by calling some, and emailing others, and viewing others online, I was able to establish how many were able to take bedridden stroke patients with dementia. This reduced the prospective homes to about 20. I called all of those and asked if there were any current vacancies. This dropped the number to six. By making enquiries with these, I found a clear favourite, and I asked if I could call in for a visit.

Heather and I set off the next Saturday morning, and we were welcomed with a warm smile and the chance of a cup of tea.

'The kettle's just boiled,' said Steve, the head nurse.

I have always believed in first impressions about people, and I think I have been right more times than I have been wrong. I liked Steve the moment we met, he smiled in a very natural, unaffected way, and somehow I just knew he was good at his job; he made a great cup of tea at the drop of a hat, too.

He took his time showing us around; there was no hurry, no rushing from room to room, and he made no effort to disguise the home's less than adequate paintwork.

'This place used to have a bad reputation,' he said. 'The people who ran it were more interested in the money than they were in the people. They never spent a penny on the place.' We looked at the faded paint, peeling off the walls in patches here and there. 'But they've gone now, and I'm going to turn it around,' he said.

I could tell he meant it.

An elderly couple passed us in the corridor, a man in his 80s, I'd say, and a woman in her 90s; they were each on Zimmer frames, but they seemed to be racing, and they were laughing and joking with each other as they inched into the day room.

'The damn programme will be finished by the time we get there!' said the old man, and the woman screeched with laughter.

'The whole place needs re-decorating,' said Steve. 'I've applied for the funds to have it done. But I promise you your mum will want for nothing here, she will be well looked-after.'

He looked me straight in the eye as he spoke, and I believed him. It's not paintwork that makes a home successful, it's the professionalism and dedication of the people who work there. The most beautiful décor means nothing if the staff don't care. This place was a bit run-down, but it had people like Steve in it and that made all the difference.

'What kind of music does she like?' he asked. It was a question I had never been asked before by anyone at any nursing home.

I smiled, as I thought about the Irish band at home. 'She likes Irish band music,' I said.

'I have a spare music centre in the closet,' said Steve. 'I'll find her a tape, we can set it up in her room.'

I was touched. It was this kind of little inexpensive thoughtfulness that made a proper home.

When Heather and I left, we both felt certain that this, at last, was the right place for mum. We chatted light-heartedly all the way home in the car, sure and certain we had made the right decision.

She was discharged from George Eliot on the Wednesday of the following week. On the Wednesday evening, Steve called me.

'Your mum is settled in fine,' he said. 'I put that spare music centre into her room, and I've got her some Irish music tapes. She's listening to them now. She's really enjoying them, she's smiling a lot.'

I felt a lump come into my throat.

'Thank you so much, Steve,' I said. I was genuinely grateful.

Four days later, he called again.

'I'm sorry to tell you that your mum has had another stroke,' he said. 'She's been rushed back to George Eliot. She's in intensive care there. I'm *so* sorry.'

27. Third Stroke

THIS NEWS CAME like a bombshell. Of all the cruel tricks to be played on mum, this was the worst. Just when she had found a place to see out the rest of her days in comfort, with people who would look after her properly and let her pass the time away listening to her favourite music, she had been allowed only four short days of peace before it was all taken away from her again.

We went back to the hospital that evening with hearts as heavy and as numb as if they were made of iron.

Mum was in the intensive care ward with the curtain drawn around her bed. All the usual stuff was there again – NIL BY MOUTH, the old tubes, the blue plastic mask. She gasped and wheezed for every breath, and the pink flush had once more disappeared from her face, to be replaced by that awful, pale grey colour that is never seen in a healthy human being.

We sat by her bedside that evening, wondering how she found the strength to carry on like this.

'She's a fighter,' observed Heather, shaking her head.

This time, there was no recognition of her surroundings at all. When mum briefly opened her eyes it was to stare straight up at the ceiling; she never moved her head to the left or to the right, never acknowledged anyone's voice, and never looked in any direction except straight up. Each breath was a battle, requiring effort and concentration. There was no strength left in her for anything or anyone else.

Both Heather and I knew the end was not far away now. Everyone knew. Again we sat down by her bedside to wait.

I took still more time off work, and stayed several nights a week sitting in the chair by her bedside, waking and falling asleep throughout each nightly vigil. There was never any sign of change. It had taken mum three months to recover from the devastating effects of the second stroke, and I didn't think she had three months of that kind of energy left inside her.

I was sitting there a few days later when the consultant came to see me again.

'We need to take some instructions from you, as the next of kin,' he said. 'There may come a time when your mum may stop breathing, she could lapse into unconsciousness, or her heart could stop. We need to know what you would like us to do if circumstances like that should occur in the near future.'

'What do you mean?' I asked.

I must have sounded so stupid. Now, it's obvious what he was telling me, but at the time I really didn't understand.

He put it more simply. 'Do you want us to try and revive her, or not?'

Then I understood.

'Your mum has very little quality of life now,' he explained. 'There will be no improvement and no recovery, I am sure. So should there be a serious lapse in her condition from where she is now, what would you like us to do?'

I knew the word I wanted to say, but to finally speak it out loud was to admit at last that all traces of hope were finally gone, and we had all accepted as much. A silence fell between us that was intense. He waited for an answer, and I was afraid to speak it. In the end I gave him the word that would both seal mum's fate, and offer her a release from all of this at long last.

'Nothing,' I said.

He nodded and left.

We were sitting in a local steak house one afternoon, a few days later, having a quiet meal. The events of the past week had taken their toll on the both of us, and we decided to go out and try to relax for a change.

The steaks had only just arrived when Heather's mobile telephone rang. She simply replied, 'Yes, okay,' and ended the call.

'That was the George Eliot,' she said. 'Your mum's just taken a turn for the worse. We have to get there within the next 20 minutes.'

We shot up from the table, paid for the untouched meal and ran into the car park.

By the time we got to the ward, 20 minutes had almost elapsed.

The curtains were drawn around mum's bed again, and I could hear her fighting for every breath outside in the corridor. Each time she inhaled, her head moved slightly backwards and her chest arched, as though it was causing her a supreme effort. She continued to fight like this for the next five-and-a-half hours, until sheer physical exhaustion overtook her, and she fell into a deep sleep where her breathing noticeably quietened, and seemed to come a little easier.

Heather went home to get some sleep. I stayed with mum all night again.

In the morning the consultant came to see her, and he shook his head in quiet disbelief.

'She's a tough lady,' he said, more to himself, I think, than to me.

'She always has been,' I replied.

He shook his head again, and walked away.

I took the following day off work and stayed with mum until late the following evening. She had now exceeded by a day-and-a-half the 20 minutes the hospital thought would see out the end of her life. The crisis seemed to have passed, and she was sleeping and breathing normally again.

I went home to get some sleep.

Heather and I were having a late supper, we were chatting about the bills, and other mundane stuff that seems to take up so much of life, when the telephone rang. Heather answered it. I knew immediately what had happened when her voice broke and she started to cry before she replaced the receiver.

She put her arms around me and told me that mum had died peacefully in her sleep only five minutes ago. Suddenly the bills didn't seem to matter any more. Death puts everything else into perspective.

28. A Quiet Farewell

WE MADE THE final journey to the hospital in silence, Heather and I. This time there was no need for speed, no panic, no sense that we might be too late: we knew we were too late. We parked the car as usual, and walked down the winding corridors of the hospital's thoroughfares, until we came at last to the intensive care unit. The nurses at the reception desk smiled kindly at us, and one of them came over.

'We're all very sorry,' she said.

'Thank you,' I replied, 'and thank you for all you've done for my mum over the months.'

'It was a pleasure,' she replied. 'Your mum was no trouble at all, she was lovely.'

Heather put her arm through mine and we leaned gently against each other.

'There is some paperwork I have to go through with you,' resumed the nurse. 'It can wait though, if you're not up to it right now.'

'No, I understand,' I said. 'What is it?'

The nurse started to explain several sheets of paper to me, but I wasn't really listening. I signed them at the bottom without knowing what I was signing for.

'*Never sign anything without reading it first,*' my dad had always said to me.

'Can we see her?' I asked.

'Of course,' replied the nurse.

The curtains were drawn around mum's bed. When we passed through them, the first thing I noticed was the silence. Mum had been fighting noisily for every breath; now there was no breath, and no noise. She lay on her back with her neck arched and her mouth open, in the same posture I had seen her when the battle for every breath was raging. I kissed her one last time on the forehead.

'Goodnight, mum,' I whispered.

Beside her bed were her personal things, gathered up from the windowsill – her toothbrush, shampoo, a bottle of moisturiser. In collecting her things, someone had moved a small glass vase of flowers which had belonged to the lady in the opposite bed, and had placed them on top of mum's radiator. Flowers on the little girl's radiator: *How wonderfully fitting*, I thought.

We left mum's unused toiletries with the staff to be distributed to the patients as they saw fit. We thanked the nurses, and left the hospital for the last time.

When we got home, I telephoned my Aunt Ellen in Ireland. She cried, and said it was for the best, and asked me to let her know when the funeral would be, so she could come over.

The following day, I started to go through mum's private papers. I felt like I was betraying her, somehow; that these were none of my business. But if I didn't do it, who else was there? I found her will, where she left all her jewellery to my daughter Rebecca, and a small sum of money to my son, Daniel. The house came to me, and that was it.

I stood there, looking around. It is surprising what we gather about us in a lifetime. In every corner of the house there was a reminder of mum; some little ornament, a book, a picture. We leave the tracks of our footsteps through life with the knick-knacks we leave behind.

Within a week, those who needed to know had been told and an entire life which had taken over 80 years to unfold was legally wrapped up, tied with a bow and marked, 'Finished.'

We arranged the funeral for the following week at the crematorium in Coventry, and at 10 o'clock, on a cold, drizzly, November morning we gathered to pay our respects. Rebecca and Daniel were there, along with Heather's three grown-up daughters, who had never met mum but who came with their partners to show support for me. I was very touched by that. My old mates came with their partners, and the rest of mum's family from Dublin, as promised.

It was a quiet farewell, but I think my dad would have approved.

The service was calm and dignified, and when it was over, we trooped back out into the cold and drizzle to gather and reminisce.

There was a line of wreaths and flowers beside a wall outside the chapel, and we all went along reading the inscriptions in turn. There was one from Steve at mum's last home; she had only been with him for four days, and yet he had taken the trouble. I was sorry she had not been under his care from the very beginning.

We laid on some food and drink at our place in Nuneaton, and a few people came back. By the early evening, everyone had gone, and the funeral formalities were over.

The following Saturday morning, Heather and I waited at St. Paul's cemetery in Holbrooks for the funeral director to arrive. There was just the two of us.

It may seem completely inappropriate here, but I will now tell you a funny story. I have to really, as it will explain why my father's ashes had been under our hall table since he had died five years earlier, and why he was only being buried with mum that morning.

One day, just a week before he died, dad had called my mother and me to the armchair in the conservatory where he used to sit on nice afternoons. 'When I die,' he said, 'I want you to take me home.'

My dad had been born in Dublin in 1921, and had died in Coventry in 2002; he was 81, and had lived in Coventry since he was 30. But despite the fact that he had been in England longer than in Ireland, he always talked of Ireland as 'home'. 'I think I might go home for a holiday this year,' he'd say, meaning he'd go to Dublin. So that November afternoon, we knew he meant he wanted to be buried in Dublin.

'Oh, don't be saying things like that, Benny!' exclaimed mum. 'You know talk like that upsets me.'

'Now, Rose,' he replied, 'these things have to be said. It's just a fact of life, that's all, and I would like you to take me home when the time comes. Promise me now, Rose.'

Mum promised him, and changed the subject. She had no intention of burying him anywhere outside Coventry, but she didn't want to talk about dying, either, so she just agreed to anything he wanted to shut him up. I knew mum and her little ways, but so did my dad.

'I mean it,' he went on. 'Martin, I'm trusting you to make sure your mother takes me home. Now, will you promise me that, son?'

I said that I promised, and he finally let the matter drop.

When he did pass away, I reminded mum of our last promise to him, and booked her a return flight to Dublin. I couldn't get the time off work, so she was going on her own.

'You can spend a few weeks with Aunty Ellen,' I said. 'See to dad as soon as you get there, and then have a little holiday. It will do you good.'

'That sounds like a good idea,' agreed mum.

A few days later, we drove out to Birmingham airport. Dad was in a little square wooden box with a brass plaque on the lid – he had been cremated, obviously – and mum intended to take him on the aeroplane as hand luggage. She was carrying his casket in a Sainsbury's plastic carrier bag, and, so that she didn't draw attention to it and upset the other passengers, she had placed a bag of carrots on top of him.

'I wish you were coming with me, son,' she said, as I kissed her goodbye at the departure gate.

'It can't be helped, mum,' I said. 'Have a nice flight. Call me when you get there.'

I drove home from the airport and waited for her to call upon landing at Dublin. The flight only took 40 minutes, and because I knew the flight number, the touch-down time, how long it would take to clear customs and so on, I had a pretty good idea when I could expect her to call.

Right on the button, the telephone rang. It was mum, but she was hysterical and in floods of tears.

'Oh son, I can't find your daddy anywhere!' she wailed.

'Well, he can't have gone far, can he?' I said, laughing.

'Don't be making jokes at a time like this!' shouted mum. 'I'm very upset!'

'Well, how could you have lost him?' I asked.

'I don't know!' she wailed. 'One minute he was there, and then next minute he was gone. Where can he be?'

'Is Aunty Ellen with you?' I asked. I knew I would get more sense from my aunty.

'She is. Do you want to speak to her, son?' sobbed mum.

'Yes, put her on.'

'Hello Martin, this is your Aunty Ellen.'

'Hello, Aunty Ellen.'

'Oh Martin, what in the name of God is she like?' asked my aunt.

'I don't know,' I replied.

'Are you sure she had your daddy on the plane, Martin?'

'I left her at the departure gate, he was with her then.'

'Martin, would you ever check at Birmingham airport to see if anyone has found your daddy?' asked Aunt Ellen.

She made it sound like he had recently developed a habit of wandering off.

'Okay, I will,' I agreed. 'Just go back to your house and I'll call you there later.'

'Right-oh, Martin, we'll do that, God Bless.'

The line went dead.

I got into the car and drove back to Birmingham airport. I thought I would start with security.

'Has anyone handed in a funeral casket and a bag of carrots?' I asked the slightly startled security guard.

'I'll check,' he said.

He whispered into his shoulder radio. I couldn't hear what he said as he wandered a few paces away when he made the enquiry. He came back to me after a couple of minutes.

'As a matter of fact, they have,' he said. 'You can pick them up at the supervisor's office.' He gave me the directions.

I took dad's casket and the carrots back to our house and called Aunty Ellen's house in Dublin.

'Oh, that's great news!' said Aunty Ellen. 'I'll tell your mum. Where was he?'

'Someone must have found him and handed him in,' I replied.

'Was he in Lost Property?' she said. Like it really mattered.

'No, the security people had him,' I said.

'Oh that's good,' she said.

Mum stayed two weeks with her sister and had a wonderful holiday, and never got round to taking him back – it was shortly after this that she began the first stages of her Alzheimer's. For five years, dad had stayed put under the small telephone table in our hallway at home. Which is why, on the morning of mum's burial, we interred my dad at the same time. I knew I'd not fulfilled my promise to him; but I also knew he'd have wanted to be here, with mum.

The funeral director's van drew up next to us at the cemetery.

He got out holding mum's casket, and Heather and I got out holding dad's. The three of us walked slowly down the short path to the small open graveside.

'Do you want to say a few words?' asked the funeral director.

I felt as though I should, but the words just wouldn't come.

I shook my head.

'Shall I say a short prayer?' asked the funeral director.

'Yes please,' I said. Suddenly a lump had come into my throat, and I knew my voice was shaking.

We placed the two small wooden caskets, side-by-side into the cold, damp hole. The funeral director read a passage from the bible that was very moving (and which I sadly cannot remember now), and when he was finished, he said: 'I'll leave you to your thoughts,' and slowly walked away.

Heather and I stood there, arm-in-arm by the side of the hole in the ground. I looked down into the cavity to read the brass plaques on the two caskets for the last time.

BERNARD SLEVIN
BORN 21/6/1921
DIED 15/11/2002

ROSE MARY SLEVIN
BORN 8/9/1925
DIED 15/11/2007

I kept looking at the dates of death on the two plaques. It hadn't hit me before, but Mum had died exactly five years to the day after dad; I wondered if she had been waiting, fighting for every last breath until the right day came, when she could finally let go. I wondered if dad had been waiting for her.

I stood up from the graveside and thought about mum. I thought about the forest of my socks pinned to the ceiling and walls. I thought about the giant Christmas goose. I thought about Michael and the Irish band, and how they had played many a ballad and jig for mum, transporting her back on those soft Celtic airs to a more romantic time in her youth. I thought about the friends she had made on her sad and lonely journey: Captain John, who believed he still lived on a boat; the old fighter pilot, whom she had wanted to marry; Joyce, who had believed that everyone else was a bit gone in the head; the whistling woman, who had just stopped whistling one day; the old lady who had been dragged out of bed by her feet; and the man in the grey macintosh.

I thought about all the letters I had written for her. I thought about the innocent delight she had derived from our old and bedraggled Christmas tree. I thought about Bruno and his shaved bum.

And I couldn't help but smile.

Then in my mind's eye I saw her, the little girl, standing on the other side of the tiny grave. She was six years old or so, in a pretty pink dress with a matching bow in her hair, and clasping an armful of much-loved teddies. She smiled at me, with that innocent and open confidence only children can have, when their entire lives stretch out before them like a blank canvas, when all things in life are yet possible and the savage storms of Life and Time have not yet touched their little empires. When all is as it seems, and the discoveries of life are the enchantments of a single, sunny afternoon. There she was, little Rose, bejewelled with the fantastic, pure magic of childhood, which swirled and flowed around her like a visible cloud. There she was, unconfused, innocent, and receptive to all the joys of living; totally unconcerned for the future, and focused entirely on the present, as all happy children the world over should be. Here before me was Rose, the little girl who in the fullness of time would grow up to be my mother. Here was the little girl, shining and new, before old age had robbed her of her reason, and the vicious sneak thief, Alzheimer's, had stolen away her hope, and her future, and had left her alone, crying and frightened in the darkness.

Then she smiled again, and waved; and she turned, and was gone.

The Little Girl in the Radiator was free at last.

Last Word

So, that's it: this was my story – or, more accurately, it was my mother's story.

The true tale of one, simple Irishwoman's battle with a disease which robbed her of everything she had; ultimately, it even robbed her of her own self. If a loved one dies of cancer, or of any other wasting disease, the patient remains right up to her final breath who she was; her habits, her personality, her likes and dislikes all remain unaltered by the disease which is killing her, because it ravages only her body. With Alzheimer's, even the last vestige of who and what she is and was is eroded, until at the end there is nothing left, inside or outside, of the person we knew and loved.

At the time of writing, 25 million people in the world have Alzheimer's disease, and that figure increases every year. If we assume for the sake of the argument that, on average, each one of those patients has a circle of only four other family members who are trying to care for them, then as you read this there are over 100 million people in the world directly affected by a disease that no-one seems to be doing very much about.

If you are now, or find yourself in the future to be, one of that legion of carers, then this is my advice to you.

Remember always, that no matter what mad thing they may say, or no matter what crazy thing they may do, there is always a reason behind it. When my mother spoke and interacted with the little girl in the radiator, she was really only trying to explain to the outside world how she felt about a disease which she could not understand nor express to the rest of us. When she went through the recurring drama of constantly locking me out of the house, she was only reacting in an external way to an inner insecurity, caused by the confusion and vulnerability she felt in her daily life. When she told me wild stories of sinking ships and crashing planes, she was only reciting the dramas she had seen on the television earlier that day; and when she told me she lived in a house with a green kitchen floor, she was only describing the house of her childhood, as her mind rewound like a cassette tape, spooling backwards to her infancy.

So bear with them, and try to understand, even when your patience is tested to its human limits; try to see the humour in it, for humour there always is, and if you can laugh, then you can carry on.

Dealing with a loved one who has Alzheimer's is rather like trying to peel an onion with your bare hands; each time you tear away a layer, you find there is yet another one underneath, and the more you peel the layers away, and the closer you get to the core, the more it makes you want to cry.

Ironically, you may well find that you have the more difficult time with your loved one in the early stages of the disease, rather than later. Shortly after diagnosis, when their mental faculties are sufficient that they can understand that they have the condition, they know what that means; they may become very unhappy, tearful and depressed. In the latter stages, they don't know they have it; they have lost their short-term memory to a greater or lesser degree (everyone's different), and they may well think there is nothing wrong with them. You will have to cope with both stages.

However, there are now Alzheimer's societies everywhere, and no matter where on earth you happen to live, there is a society somewhere near you. All are readily found on the internet or via your doctor; do contact them as early as possible, as soon as the disease is diagnosed, and do not be too proud to accept their help; they can make a huge difference to your quality of life, and that of your loved one. With 100 million people spread across the face of this planet affected directly by Alzheimer's, you cannot be alone; there is a huge support group of volunteers out there for you. I did not know any of this when I cared for my mum; the support was not widely publicised. But if you have read this book, well, it doesn't have to be the same for you.

I suppose the best you can do for them is simply to continue to love them. As their condition slowly worsens over time, and their memory and focus begins to recede through their life, they will tell you of incidents which may be unknown to you, and parts of your own family history which had been unknown to you will slowly become revealed; this can be fascinating, so do listen. Involve every member of your family in the care of the patient if you can; it is not your problem alone, so ask for the responsibility to be shared – you will need a break. Do involve your local Social Services: it's one of the things they exist for.

Everyone has their limits, and one day you will realise, with painful certainty and resignation, that you have reached yours. The day will surely come when you are no longer able to look after the patient at home. This could be for a number of reasons. Perhaps your working patterns change and you will no longer be at home, so they will be left to their own devices for too long. Perhaps you will need to go away from home for extended periods, travel with your career, or just for a vacation, and you cannot realistically take the patient with you. Perhaps you simply feel that you can no longer cope; there is no shame in admitting this. When this moment is reached, and it will come, you will have to find a nursing home. Your local Social Services or the internet should be able to provide you with a list of suitable places within a reasonable distance. You will want to find homes within a reasonable radius, so that you can call in regularly. Please be aware that all these homes are not the same, and choose carefully; visit them all; take into account such things as their weekly fees, and how much help you can get towards the costs. Are they comfortable? Do they serve proper meals? What are the other residents like? Could your family member make friends there? Do the staff treat the patients as numbers, or people? What are the laundry, and hairdressing, and medical services like? Is the place generally clean and tidy? Don't be afraid to ask the most searching of questions, and make sure you speak to the manager, in depth, before you commit your loved one to one of these places.

As Alzheimer's rolls back the rug of their memory, and all inside the roll is lost forever, there may come a time when they forget who you are. My mum thought Heather was my ex-wife, and that I was her brother – until, at the end, she didn't know me at all. To be expunged from your mother's consciousness can be heart-breaking. It feels as if all that has gone before between you, all the good times and shared experiences, now counts for nothing. But that doesn't really matter. What does is that you still love them, and they still love you, somewhere deep and forgotten. Remind them, tell them about the good times you have shared; you can remember for the both of you.

God bless and good luck,
Martin Slevin.

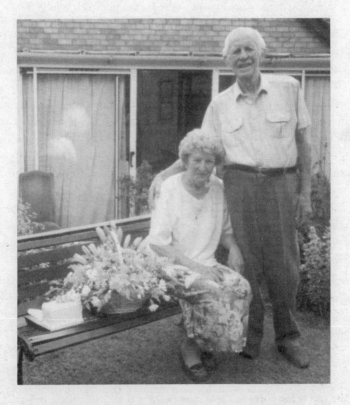

Rose and Bernard Slevin, mum and dad
Rest in peace

A Few Interesting Facts

The following information refers specifically to the United Kingdom; however, European and world figures are very similar percentage wise if extrapolated through any national population.

The number of people with dementia in the U.K. has been estimated by applying percentage figures to the known population in 2005:

England: 574,717
Northern Ireland: 15,850
Scotland: 56,106
Wales: 36,924
Total number of people with dementia in the U.K. 683,597

The documented age ranges for dementia are:

40-64 years: 1 in 1400
65-69 years: 1 in 100
70-79 years: 1 in 25
80-95 years: 1 in 6
95+ years: 1 in 3

It is estimated that by 2021 there will be 940,000 people with dementia in the U.K. This figure is expected to rise to over 1,700,000 by the year 2051; 1 in 14 people over 65 years of age, and 1 in 6 people over 80 years of age have one form or another of dementia.

Alzheimer's disease is the most common form of dementia. The proportions of those with different forms of dementia can be broken down as follows:

Alzheimer's disease (AD): 62%
Vascular dementia (VaD): 17%

Mixed dementia (AD & VaD): 10%
Dementia with Lewy bodies: 4%
Fronto-temporal dementia: 2%
Parkinson's dementia: 2%
Other dementia: 3%

Dementia is fairly rare among people under 65. However, there are 15,000 currently documented cases of young people with dementia in the U.K. The actual number may be as much as three times this figure, because the reported numbers of young cases are based on referrals to Social Services, while many young people with the disease do not seek professional help in the early stages.

Two thirds of people with dementia are women.

The proportion of people with dementia doubles for every 5-year age group.

One third of all people over 95 have dementia.

The financial cost of dementia to the U.K. is £17 billion a year; family carers for people with dementia save the U.K. £6 billion per year.

Two thirds of people with dementia live in the community, only one third live in care homes; 64% of people living in care homes have dementia.

Only 2% of medical research funding is allocated to Alzheimer's; £11 per patient per year is allocated to research funding for Alzheimer's, compared to £289 per patient per year for cancer.

Every 71 seconds someone in the U.K. develops Alzheimer's.

There are over 5 million people with dementia in Europe. And over 5 million people with dementia in the United States. There are at least

24 million people with dementia in the world; by 2025 there will be 34 million people with dementia in the world.

No-one knows what causes it.

Alzheimer's Society (United Kingdom, except Scotland)
Devon House
58 St Katharine's Way
London
E1W 1LB
Tel: 020 7423 3500
Helpline: 0845 300 0336
Email: enquiries@alzheimers.org.uk
Web: www.alzheimers.org.uk

Alzheimer Scotland – Action on Dementia
Tel: 0131 243 1453
Helpline: 0808 808 3000
Email: alzheimer@alzscot.org
Web: www.alzscot.org

Sick Notes / **Dr Tony Copperfield**

(ppbk, £8.99)

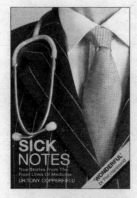

WELCOME TO the bizarre world of Tony Copperfield, family doctor. He spends his days fending off anxious mums, elderly sex maniacs and hopeless hypochondriacs (with his eyes peeled for the odd serious symptom). The rest of his time is taken up sparring with colleagues, battling bureaucrats and banging his head against the brick walls of the NHS.

If you've ever wondered what your GP is really thinking - and what's actually going on behind the scenes at your surgery - *SICK NOTES* is for you.

'A wonderful book, funny and insightful in equal measure'
– *Dr Phil Hammond (Private Eye's 'MD')*

'Copperfield is simply fantastic, unbelievably funny and improbably wise… everything he writes is truer than fact'
– *British Medical Journal*

'Original, funny and an incredible read' – *The Sun*

Tony Copperfield is a Medical Journalist of the Year, has been shortlisted for UK Columnist of the Year many times and writes regularly for *The Times* and other media.

**From all good bookshops, online from
www.mondaybooks.com or via 01455 221752.
All of our titles are also available as eBooks from amazon.co.uk**

A Paramedic's Diary / **Stuart Gray**

(ppbk, £7.99)

STUART GRAY is a paramedic dealing with the worst life can throw at him. *A Paramedic's Diary* is his gripping, blow-by-blow account of a year on the streets – 12 rollercoaster months of enormous highs and tragic lows. One day he'll save a young mother's life as she gives birth, the next he might watch a young girl die on the tarmac in front of him after a hit-and-run. A gripping, entertaining and often amusing read by a talented new writer.

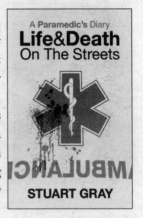

As heard on BBC Radio 4's Saturday Live and BBC Radio 5 Live's Donal McIntyre Show and Simon Mayo

In April 2010, Stuart Gray was named one of the country's 'best 40 bloggers' by *The Times*

Wasting Police Time / PC David Copperfield

(ppbk, £7.99)

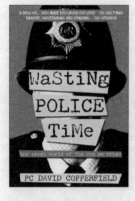

The fascinating, hilarious and best-selling inside story of the madness of modern policing. A serving officer - writing deep under cover - reveals everything the government wants hushed up about life on the beat.

'Very revealing' – *The Daily Telegraph*

'Passionate, important, interesting and genuinely revealing' – *The Sunday Times*

'Graphic, entertaining and sobering' – *The Observer*

'A huge hit... will make you laugh out loud' – *The Daily Mail*

'Hilarious... should be compulsory reading for our political masters' – *The Mail on Sunday*

'More of a fiction than Dickens' – *Tony McNulty MP, former Police Minister*

(On a BBC *Panorama* programme about PC Copperfield, McNulty was later forced to admit that this statement, made in the House of Commons, was itself inaccurate)